*A New Map
to a Healthy Gut
&Vibrant Life*

GUT
TRUTH

KARLENE
GEORGIADIS

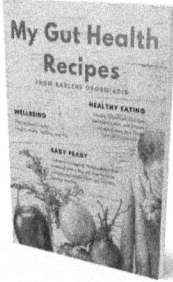

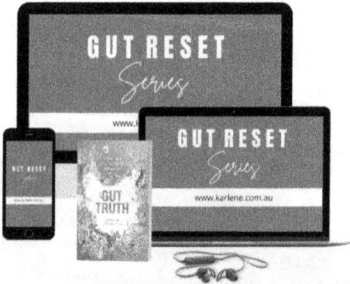

*A New Map
to a Healthy Gut
&Vibrant Life*

GUT
TRUTH

KARLENE
GEORGIADIS

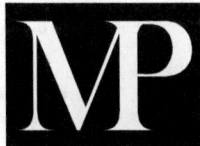

M̄P

Mind Potential Publishing
by *The Potentialist*

Author: Karlene Georgiadis
Title: Gut Truth
ISBN Paperback: 978-922380-53-1
ISBN Kindle: 978-1-922380-55-5

Author website: www.karlene.com.au

A catalogue record for this
book is available from the
National Library of Australia

Category: Health | Nutrition
Publisher: Mind Potential Publishing
Division of Mind Design Centre Pty Ltd. www.mindpotentialpublishing.com

Cover design and internal art by: Narelle Craven Logozoo
https://logozoo.com.au
Author Photography by: Adrienne Dillon www.littleblackrabbit.net
Book Formatting by: Narelle Ellis NGirl Design: www.ngirldesign.com.au

DEDICATION

To my two beautiful children Nathan and
Emily for their patience and support and love.

And to my mother, Hiltrud, for asking me
the right questions that led me to my own
answers, as I now do this daily in my work.
Bless you Mum

Karlene, xo

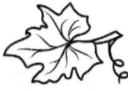

CONTENTS

FOREWORD

When I studied naturopathy in the late 1980s, we were taught that 'all diseases begin in the gut' despite the fact there was little in the scientific literature to support this hypothesis. In the past two decades following innovative technologies and mapping of the human genome, the volume of research dedicated to the microbiome and its impact on animal and human health has taken centre stage, as evident by the thousands of publications and numerous journals dedicated to this field. Much of this knowledge sits idly in journals given it can take up to 17 years to go from scientific discovery to clinical practice. As the magnitude of this discovery trickles into the health industry, a small but dedicated number of clinicians are challenging the status quo, thinking beyond their training, spending years listening to their patients, and hundreds or even thousands of hours of their own time attending lectures to help their patients. Karlene Georgiadis is one such clinician. Her dedication to her patients and dogged determination to get to the root cause(s) has discovered that your poo provides an incredible snapshot of your health which is the outcome of your genes, lifestyle and environmental factors.

Almost half of the adult population are diagnosed with at least one chronic disease and, over the years most end up on a longlist of medications. This polypharmacy approach frequently results in addictions and more often than not, negatively impacts one's physical and mental wellbeing. It certainly negatively impacted my father's health (and my parent's relationship) following his Parkinson's Disease diagnosis and subsequent addiction to over a hundred tablets per day. Is this acceptable? I think not. Is there a better way? YES!

Regardless of your state of health or diagnosis, your stool reveals your unique story and the perfect snapshot of your health. More importantly, it provides the key steps you need to take to improve your health and vitality. Karlene's approach to gut health, addresses how we can positively feed and balance our microbiota and take back control of our health. The book is brimming with real-life stories of people who have faced the kinds of challenges you face and how they gained great health. Having presented at medical conferences in Environmental Medicine both in Australia and abroad, I can personally advocate that Karlene digs deeper into the story of gut health than any other gut health book I've read. She is willing to get down and talk dirty and empower you to love and observe your stool as a gateway to good health. This engaging and thought-provoking, yet easy to read book will have you running to the phone to get your stool tested. It certainly did for me!

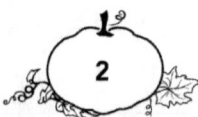

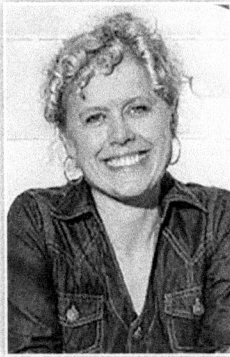

Nicole Bijlsma

Best-Selling Author & Public Figure

PhD (pending), N.D.
BHScAc(Hons.), Grad.Dip.OHS.
Dip. Building Biology,
IICRC Mould Remediator

www.buildingbiology.com.au

Nicole Bijlsma is a building biologist, bestselling author (Healthy Home Healthy Family), researcher and CEO of the Australian College of Environmental Studies (est.1999). Nicole is the founder of the Building Biology movement in Australia which was created to educate people about the health hazards in the built environment. Nicole has lectured at tertiary institutions for over 30 years, has published in peer reviewed journals and is regularly consulted by the media to discuss mould, electromagnetic fields and toxic chemicals, and lectures in Australia and abroad about environmental health issues.

INTRODUCTION
– SHOW DON'T TELL

I am overjoyed to receive emails from patients telling me they now feel great, or they are relieved to have avoided needing a colostomy bag or even that they feel that 'I saved their life'. That they feel free of their crippling symptoms, free to live their best life. I'm so humbled to read their emails.

But I'm not a life-saver. I am a solution-finder. I find the solution within your gut. In fact, I find that solution in the last place any person wants to look: your poo!

Yup, buried in your poo lies a solution so transformative and powerful that it saves lives. Don't worry, I do the dirty work. All you have to do is start realizing that within your gut lies your own unique healing solution.

Every patient who finds me has already seen genuinely caring physicians, dieticians, nutritionists, naturopaths and healers who did their best to bring about better health. Many patients have become desperate for a miracle because nothing else got the level of results they wanted.

And that's exactly what I do, but it's not my miracle cure made from secret herbs and nutrients. It's your very own innate ability to heal, which has been lying dormant in your gut waiting for an opportunity to be activated. I help patients access the truth

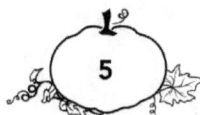

from within their gut and achieve incredible health potential and freedom.

There have been many times when a new patient has confided in me and told me they feel so exhausted after years of trying to 'crack the code' on their health, many even tell me they find it difficult to believe they can ever feel well again.

I don't waste time trying to TELL someone who has lost hope in their body's ability to heal, I instead SHOW them. There's nothing like feeling well again to inspire the biggest cynic. Best of all, when I guide patients to their own 'code' and their body begins to heal itself, they get their lives back, and I get heartfelt emails in my inbox to start my day with joy!

- No longer does Joyce need to cancel a nursing shift because she can't muster enough energy to shower let alone get through an entire shift.
- Nor Cameron, who can't get off the toilet long enough to make it out of the driveway, let alone sit in peak hour traffic.

Imagine that Joyce and Cameron no longer wonder IF they will ever feel better, because they KNOW how great it feels to be healthy!

As you read this book you will hear real life stories of irritable bowel syndrome (IBS), sexual dysfunction, auto-immune conditions, you name it, and each case will involve a unique treatment with one

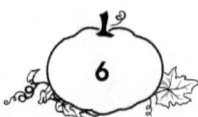

thing in common: The body only heals when you activate your gut's unique healing solution.

Let's get started on your unique healing code to fix your gut.

Until now you have understandably been consumed by your suffering. I get it.

But right here, right now, choose to be done with suffering and instead decide consciously and willingly to align yourself with health and vitality, these are your birthright.

I need you to set aside your fears and doubts and stop doing what doesn't work. By doing this you can get out of the way of your own healing and start to feel empowered, vital and strong.

I know that your gut has phenomenal healing power.

By taking specific steps, you will establish a miraculous gut forest that grows your body's own cure. A forest so small that it can't be seen by the naked eye but so vast that it will change your physiology from symptomatic to super-cala-fragilistic-expialadotious!

What is the starting point for your gut's healing power?

Your Poo of course!

The last place that most people want to start is the first step to their natural and lasting solution. Let's go!

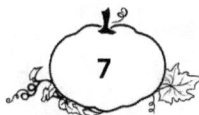

INTRODUCTION

Why poo? Really??

Your poo tells the story of your unique pathway to sickness and health.

In a clinical setting I use the word "stool." It's more professional, clinical and sounds nicer. Some patients laugh and call it 'their shit', but more often I make it conversational by using the word "poo."

This makes the topic seem more childlike and friendly, doesn't it? But at the end of the day, do you know what I hear people say most often about me and the work I do?

They say *"Karlene really knows her shit!!"*

When did we stop talking about shit? I know many of you are secretly fascinated with the topic and want to come out and talk openly about it. Some not so, and that's ok, many of us were perhaps shamed over poo accidents during childhood.

Your gut gurgles, cramps, stitches, fascinates and worries you. Nausea, burping, reflux, heartburn, bloating and farting. These all may feature in your day. For some people, they'd swear until they were blue in the face that they don't do any of these things. Here's the thing though – everyone is human, and we know that they do!

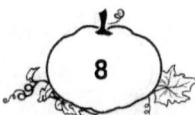

I hope I can make you just as fascinated about your poo as I am. Perhaps you want to know if your poo is good, bad, offensive, high quality or even good enough to transplant into another gut? Yes indeed, there is even a type of therapy where a 'poo transplant' occurs. The medical term for this type of procedure is a *faecal transplant*.

Perhaps you're a 'closet' poo detective, or perhaps like me, you're out there proclaiming your interest to the world. Either way, this book will be a scintillating eye opener for you. I am here to lift the veil on your poo and what it means for your health.

I outline the different types:

- [ ] The good shit
- [ ] The bad shit
- [ ] The offensive
- [ ] The super smelly rank ones!
- [ ] The sinkers
- [ ] The floaters and
- [ ] The squirters

I will tell you why your poo matters and the messages it sends you from deep inside…your gut. In this this book, I want to share with you why you should be fascinated with your poo too.

When I discuss an in-depth gut protocol with a client, it can get quite complex as the gut bacteria often dictate what your gut can and can't handle – what you can and can't digest. What will feed and what will ferment in the gut and turn into those well-known symptoms that stop the ease and flow of our daily lives. Yes, I mean, gas.

> The build-up of gas has to go somewhere. But the question is not where does it go, we kind of know that, don't we? The real question is really this: *where is the gas coming from?*

The build-up of gas is often perplexing to patients, especially when they have been working so hard to be well and eat clean and get healthy.

Many patients even diligently follow a healthy diet, but never truly account for what is happening on the inside. Inside your gut is a secret little microbiota factory and sometimes not so secret when it escapes as bottom blasts, mouth burps and general hiccupping swallows and noisy gasps.

Humans have spent a lot of time looking outside ourselves as we search for answers to life in space and what is contained in the depths of the oceans. Until recently, we largely ignored the complex universe that is within our own bodies. This universe has a huge influence on our well-being, the way we reproduce and how we age. It impacts our mood, how we think and our relationships with others.

Our gut microbiota is inextricably linked to what we eat, how we grow food and where our food comes from. It's also linked to the chemicals added to our food from the paddock to the plate, and the chemicals we add to our bodies in many different forms, including from medication, the way we were born and how we interact with all the microbes in our environment throughout life.

Microbiome/Microbiota – What's in a Name?

I notice that the words 'microbiome' and 'microbiota' appear to be used interchangeably and often to point to the same thing. However, in this book I refer to the microbiota, that is, the specific microorganisms found in an environment including bacteria, viruses and fungi.

I use microbiome to refer to the collection of microorganisms and their genes in the environment. I see it as the difference between the forest and the trees.

The microbiome is the whole of the forest with all of the trees, shrubs, animals and insects.

The microbiota are the specific trees and particular shrubs, animals and insects.

Very early in my deepest dives into the microbiota of the gut, I happily came across a talk by Dr Terry Wahls and her journey with multiple sclerosis.

Dr Wahls' protocol was a great introduction to the healing power of vegetables. She presents a protocol with a gentle phasing out of the inflammatory foods, while you build up the good stuff. It's a doable approach for anyone with autoimmunity as well as anyone wishing to improve overall gut health and health outcomes.

> Spending time at the organic greengrocer, in your garden and your kitchen is going to be time well spent investing in your health and pay back dividends over and over as you get on with living a full life.

Timing is everything and it is never too late (or too early) to start. These are new frontiers for many of us, and solving what's wrong, starts by getting to know *your* poo to achieve your own unique gut truth.

This is all about you taking responsibility for the optimal functioning of your gut and becoming your own system engineer. An engineer with knowledge and motivation to achieve optimal functioning and health of all body systems.

Who is this book for?

This book is for you, my dear friend. It's about the signals and messages your gut is sending out and what it means for you and your mood, long-term health and longevity, including:

- How to interpret these signs and how they are reflected in the quality of your poo, and of course what to do to rebalance it all.

- What to do to entirely turn your health around via your gut.

- How to stop the downward slide in your gut health and digestion, uplift your energy and return to your optimal health potential.

This book is also for anyone who:

- Has had ongoing gut symptoms for weeks, months, years, or even decades who has potentially tried many diets and ways to support digestion without long lasting relief.

- Has been struggling with gut health and symptoms of wind, bloating, burping, reflux, weight gain, loose stools, diarrhea and constipation and no matter what they have tried, has found limited relief.

- Is sick of not getting lasting answers for their digestive upsets as nothing seems to work.

- Has been diagnosed with Crohn's disease or Ulcerative Colitis and wants to be more proactive about managing their health.

- For people who cannot seem to eat anything without some sort of digestive symptoms and who are sick of trying all sort of diets and supplements without any ongoing relief.

- Has a love-hate relationship with their gut.

- Cannot work out what is wrong, no matter how hard they've tried.

- Has been diagnosed with an autoimmune condition and is seeking to take control of their health outcomes.

This book will help you to:

- Understand what to eat to reduce symptoms of bloating, wind, reflux, diarrhea, or constipation.

- Know what the optimal stool should look and feel like and achieve perfect 10 out of 10 stools every day.

- Be free from digestive pain for good.

- Improve mood via healthy gut function.

My Story

With more than 2 decades in the nutrition and naturopathic industry, I have worked with thousands of people, just like *you*, on their health journey. Over the last 16 years I have focused on this very important area of gut health and worked with advanced stool testing methods which reveal so much about *every* aspect of digestion.

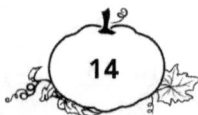

Importantly, stool testing also tells us about many other aspects of health, including brain and cognitive health, as well as immune health and the complexity of autoimmunity.

It was my own journey with chronic fatigue syndrome that led me down this path. Delving deeper into what was going on in my gut and testing myself – the way I continue to do with patients now – led to amazing health benefits. The level of recovery that I experienced was so significant and resulted in the single most important thing I did on my path to recovery.

My mission is to share the truth that there is a path to recovery. Starting as soon as you're ready for it. I want to share this with as many people as possible to show you that your biggest health mystery, that thing that you and your medical team or mental health team have tried to put a name to, has potential origins in the gut. And, importantly, that there is something that can be done to either manage it better or to even overcome it.

I have submitted and analyzed *thousands* of stool samples for investigation. This offers the patients I work with giant leaps forward in understanding their own health journey and how to interpret their own health signals. This empowers them to feel in control of that great health mystery they've been tormented by. To finally know what to do about the symptoms and how to treat the cause.

That's the map that you need to follow in order to go from ill gut health to great gut health and wellbeing.

In this book you will discover how to heal by knowing:

1. How to recognize all the signals your gut is sending you.
2. What it means when you burp a lot.
3. What causes acid reflux/heartburn and what to do about it.
4. Why you get bloated.
5. What it means when you are super farty.
6. What it means when your farts are really smelly.
7. What it means when your poo is like pebbles.
8. Or when your poo is skinny.
9. Or mushy, loose and unformed.
10. Why it matters if your poo floats.
11. How to recognize the perfect poo.
12. How to activate your gut's unique healing code.

By the end of this book, you can expect improved digestion and reduced symptoms when you put my 5 Step Process into action. When you know what your gut needs to make the perfect poo every day it's guaranteed to put a smile on your face (and mine).

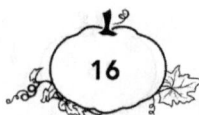

The 5 Step Process is:

Step one:	**The Symptoms**
Step two:	**The Test**
Step three:	**The Gut Protocol**
Step four:	**The Flow Check-up**
Step five:	**Your New Map to a Healthy and Vibrant Life**

Everyone needs a roadmap when it comes to health. Your gut has your unique map, but you didn't know how to read it, nor did those who have tried to help you thus far, despite of course, their best intentions.

This is your map.
And we have one basic, non-negotiable rule when it comes to maps: follow-the-map. Otherwise, you will get lost or end up going around in circles again and that's a ton of suffering you don't need.

And let's also be clear, Dr Google isn't on your map. Has Dr Google ever scared you? It's a minefield out there, with a mix of some good information, but lots of poorly researched misinformation or even bad advice which can potentially bring catastrophic outcomes.

A Map to Good Gut Health

This book is your "go to gut bible." It will help you understand the mystery and meaning of the symptoms you are experiencing, and how to address these symptoms. Let's start by tapping into the cause and opening the way for the healing to begin.

Grab yourself a notebook and make notes while reading this book to create your personalized plan, the roadmap to great gut health. This will become your path to everything you need to do to be in the best health and the best version of you.

> This is not a generic one size fits all approach, because you are not generic.

You are an individual, with your unique physiology and way of processing the environment, emotions, stress and the world. You have your own story which is part of your unique path to this very moment in time. This means that a one size fits all approach would only work if everyone else had also experienced the same story, mental, emotional and environmental influences.

If your current path got you here, then it will be a unique path that gets you to where you want to be. Besides, most of us have already tried to achieve health with a generic one size fits all approach or have previously been treated that to no avail.

If you're reading this book, chances are generic approaches haven't worked for you, but that's not your fault. You are unique and it is still possible to activate the healing within you.

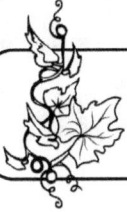

> You, your gut health, and your dietary requirements are as individual as your fingerprint.

There is no one else that needs the exact same thing you need. This book is about you finally figuring out what your gut needs to heal you so that you can thrive.

Your roadmap will empower you to move forward and begin a life-changing action-plan!

Strap yourself in! Let's get ready for a whole new level of health.

Karlene x

Chapter One

KNOW YOUR SHIT

DE-CODING INTERNAL MESSAGES

*Stories about the lies we are told, our own
inner critic, sugar carvings, IBS and self harm*

Every stool sample tells a story.

As much as I am a thorough and rigorous scientist in my work, I often feel as though I'm reading tea leaves when analyzing a stool-sample report. The mysteries reveal themselves to me, just like finding clues to a puzzle that finally makes sense.

My book is called Gut Truth because the gut doesn't lie. It is an honest reflection of not just your diet, but your lifestyle and your relationship to your own 'truth' as a human being. Changing your diet is not enough to bring about wellbeing and happiness if you are in a stressful job, surviving on poor sleep and never making time for those you love and enjoying life!

When people come to me feeling hopeless and helpless, it can be hard to imagine making changes in all of the areas and the person can become overwhelmed. I want you to know that change is always possible. It's never too late to change if the desire to do so is there. Sometimes you just know it can be better and sometimes the pain of recognizing where you are is what provides the impetus to change, even if the process of change also requires some pain.

I know from experience, and so do many of my patients, that it is better to consciously choose when and how to change. You always have a choice and lots of small changes over time will make a big difference.

Every change you make to improve your diet, will improve your wellbeing and you will be more aligned with the truth of who you

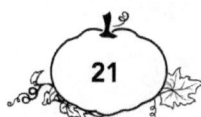

are and soon your sleep and attitude also improve! Noticing these positive changes builds into a feeling of positive momentum and greater self-confidence!

You are not just learning how to fix your gut, you will also naturally begin to respect it too! Begin by recognizing the 'gut-feeling' that you get about making changes. Deep inside there is a healing wisdom that longs to be heard. It knows the way – in fact it knows some very powerful Gut Truths!

Imagine that alongside certain foods that disagree with your gut, there may also be some beliefs and ideas that you also cannot digest. When Sally's parents divorced she was 15, she suddenly felt overwhelmed with sadness that she kept inside because she could see that her parents were stressed. Sally began a habit of eating sweets on her way home from school to distract herself from her feeling unsettled now that she had to move between two different households.

Over time Sally's gut craved more sugar and she found herself secretly eating sweets into the evening as she did her homework. Before long Sally had gained weight and became self-conscious and stressed but feeling this way now also led to more 'comfort-eating'. Without ever intending to, Sally had fallen into a vicious cycle of feeding cravings and then judging her behaviour and her body.

Her 'inner critic' said harsher comments than any of the bullies at school and in time, Sally discovered the nightmare of yo-yo dieting where desperate self-loathing led to impulsive short term weight-loss, followed by weight-gain. And repeat.

Years passed by and Sally's inner critic was the loudest voice in her mind, narrating her life-story from its singularly distorted perspective. She swallowed its lies and untruths as much as she swallowed down advice from the latest slim 'expert'. The feeling of unease that these lies cause cannot be 'digested' because it is only truth that feels peaceful, it is therefore truth that can be assimilated. Similarly, only healthy foods can be properly digested in the gut to be converted into nutrition.

> Being in Your Truth is not only good for you,
> it is one of the keys to a vibrant life.

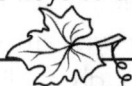

Imagine if Sally kicked the sugar habit but her inner critic still had free reign in her mind? I'm called the Poo Queen by many patients because I'm not scared of your shit. If you have experienced the pain of trauma and loss, I want to know because a symptom of these experiences is to internalize emotions and 'self-blame' and of course it is not your fault if you have been abused or victimized.

Returning to Sally's story, to use a common albeit coarse expression, she was made to 'Eat Shit' originally by the bullies and then also by her inner critic. She then internalized this and made an unconscious decision that she was a 'shit-person.' Like all of us, Sally is so much more than her weight or the diet she is trying, and she is definitely not the problem!

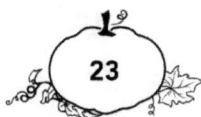

When Sally sought comfort for her emotional pain through sweets, it was simply a *symptom*, not a character flaw! She didn't lack willpower, she lacked a voice. As we will see later in the book, sugar can very quickly overgrow those sugar hungry bacteria and create a relentless wave of cravings.

> Your gut is telling you some dietary truths, but we need to listen out for the truths that sit very uncomfortably in your gut. The shit you think about yourself as true, may indeed not be true!

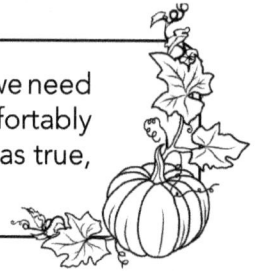

I want you to consider that when we internalize an untruth, it becomes an 'indigestible-lie', that makes us sick. Very often our eating habits and our lifestyle are closely tied to core-beliefs about not being good enough, feeling unsafe in life, not being powerful or being unlovable. This shit stinks! You deserve to see yourself as a lovable and loving human being and know that you are 'more than enough.'

We need to heal our wounds and heal our gut and in both cases the truth will set you free! Begin by changing your relationship to your inner-critic. Work on observing it, rather than automatically believing it or obeying it. Do the same with cravings - observe them rather than follow them and as your gut bacteria changes, the cravings will ease and eventually cease. Seriously! They really will!

Feed yourself an inner dialogue diet of positives and compassion. You are human, so you will sometimes make mistakes, like everyone else. Begin to practise kindness, knowing that your gut is listening!

Now, simply close your eyes and ask your gut to tell you when to begin.

Don't be afraid if it comes back with a loud, 'START NOW!'

Marjorie's Low Energy and Rapid Weight loss Story

I had the honour of helping Marjorie, a woman in her late 80s who was suffering from dreadful digestive issues. Her family were distressed, grimly watching as they saw their matriarch decline.

One of Marjorie's family members contacted me, desperate for me to help their mother. As I explained the process that could possibly be involved, they were dubious that Marjorie was capable.

I accept and respect that this path is not for everyone. It can be tough. There are a lot of changes to endure and often things get worse before they get better. However, in Marjorie's case I wondered how much worse they could get. Her symptoms were debilitating and erupted without warning.

Her symptoms featured allergies with severe coughing fits, nausea and vomiting – seemingly out of the blue. Lots of saliva would come up with air. Weight loss was rapid and as each kilogram fell away, Marjorie's energy was fading fast.

The mystery needed to be unravelled.

In Marjorie's case, more than just a stool sample was needed as the symptoms had continued for so long. I was concerned for her nutrient levels as well as her physiology so trips back to the doctor and gastroenterologist were also on the agenda.

When Marjorie's blood test results came back, I noticed there was something called a high anion gap[1]. This was the key marker that told me the truth about Marjorie's gut microbiota was part of her previously unexplained symptoms. This marker helps me to identify metabolic acidosis. The test is available through a standard blood test from your General Practitioner or licensed Physician.

Often it is the gut bacteria that are producing this acid – causing this gap to become quite high, along with other symptoms such as headache, fatigue, weakness, feeling sick in the stomach, nausea, vomiting, fast heartbeat as well as long and deep breaths. There were some key symptoms experienced by Marjorie that were pointing straight to an imbalance in her gut.

My analysis of Marjorie's microbiota revealed a bacterial imbalance, which included bacteria feeding on sugar and producing abundant amines. This was also contributing to Marjorie's allergy picture. Treatment and a change of diet was needed to suppress the overgrowth of bacteria. Also, Marjorie needed to feed the important Bacteroides that were quite low.

---

1   The anion gap is a measure of the difference between the positive ions (sodium and potassium) and the negative ions (bicarbonate and chloride) in our blood. The foods we eat, the liquids we drink and the microbiota we have directly contribute to the anion gap shown by our blood. The anion gap helps me to identify metabolic acidosis and an imbalance in the gut.

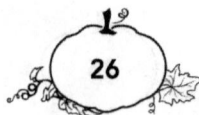

The answer to feeding our wonderful microbiota is often to increase insoluble fibers. By insoluble fibers I mean vegetable fibers including the skins and the peels from the fibrous parts of the vegetables. These are often the bits we tend to peel or cut off and throw away, but guess who needs these? Your Bacteroides do and therefore YOU do too.

For Marjorie, a change in diet to reduce acidity and supress the overgrowth of bacteria was necessary. A little slip up here and there was experienced with an immediate return of symptoms. I advised her to embrace these symptoms when they returned. A slip up served as a reminder of how good she could feel when all was going well. She began to recognize what would happen if she fell off the wagon, and that motivated her to stay on track. The slip ups started to become more and more rare.

What was also interesting was that further testing revealed some very low nutrient markers such as iron, vitamin D, and zinc. If these had stayed low, it would have hindered Marjorie's healing process. After I advised Marjorie to address these results with appropriate supplements and foods, she improved again.

The final part of the puzzle was a sneaky rolling hiatus hernia. Bingo! The hernia was the answer to why these symptoms came and went without rhyme or reason. When I consulted with the microbiologist about Marjorie's results, he was very concerned that she was well into her 80s, yet here I was making all these changes to her diet and asking her to ramp up the supplements. I answered him by saying, *"It's ok, it is her choice, she wants to do this."* And she did.

Eight weeks later when I saw Marjorie again, I saw a very different woman.

Improved energy – tick!

Marjorie said, *"I'm now able to walk three kilometres with the dog. I haven't done that for 15 years without being exhausted. Now I can do it and come home, and I still have energy."* A fantastic win for Marjorie (and the dog).

Marjorie now has the energy to go out again with friends and she can do so without the fear of the symptoms suddenly coming on. Marjorie added, *"With the hiatus hernia, I still have to be careful with food choices."*

With a hiatus hernia there are definite 'no no's' and things that you can do to ensure better digestion.

When I saw the re-energized Marjorie, I was over the moon with the amazing results. But it was Marjorie who had her quality of life back, and of course, her family, who had their adored mother back. They were all incredibly proud of the choices and effort Marjorie had made to turn her health around. This was no easy feat but imagine if she did not make these changes and the quality of her life, and the state of her health continued to decline?

Marjorie's gut healing code was waiting to be activated all along and it's always better late than never! Super-Inspirational!

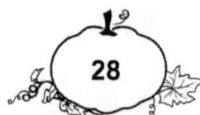

Every patient's story has its own twists and turns. Let me give you a number of insights into my own gut journey and why some aspects of my protocol have become a central part of the treatment for so many of my patients.

Insights into My Own Health Journey

I've been a naturopath for over two decades and it comes from a lifelong fascination with health. I've always been interested in what constitutes a healthy diet and how to improve the function of my body (and mind). Things like yoga, meditation, exercise, diet and sleep have always been big on my agenda.

I now understand what my body needs to stay vibrant. I know what I need to do to be able to do the things I want to do in life.

However, life does have a way of throwing curve balls. I have a sensitive constitution and prior to becoming a naturopath suffered for 20 years with symptoms of irritable bowel syndrome (IBS). In the early days, my body would crash, and I was also encumbered by chronic fatigue syndrome.

The difficulty, as many of you will know, is that these syndromes are not routinely recognized by the mainstream medical system. Some doctors will simply refuse to acknowledge they exist. Others use the term 'syndrome,' which simply refers to a collection of symptoms, but not the root cause. Even if they do acknowledge the challenges you face, some won't know what to do about the problem and often send you back out into the world again without a solution, and with little relief, let alone hope.

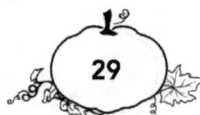

After many years, I found an Integrative Doctor who was very thorough and suggested a stool analysis. As a single mother, scraping by at the time, I must admit I was hesitant when I heard the cost of the stool test.

Initially I put off doing the test and thought I could outsmart the results by doing my own detox. Well, I detoxed and detoxed some more, and guess what? My symptoms did not magically disappear. In fact, the symptoms remained, and I became even more frustrated. I thought I was doing all the right things. I was constantly uncomfortable with awful wind and bloating. I had low energy and mood changes were also ongoing.

At this point I was frustrated with myself and everything else I had been told in the past. I even began to question some of the concepts I'd learned in college. I felt demoralized as I had followed a great diet to the letter and seen no improvements.

I finally had to surrender and decided to dive in and do the stool test.

I now love being a health detective for my patients, but it all began by getting curious about what the stool test could tell me about what was going on inside my gut and how it was affecting my day-to-day health, energy and mood.

And the results were highly specific – it was my poo! I had a typical 'fatigue pattern' and my gut microbe stool test analysis reflected a major imbalance. I learned all about the differences

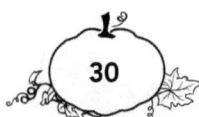

between bacteria species and how I was feeding them with what I consumed. I had no idea I had such an intricate array of residents living in my digestive system. I finally understood that their numbers and the balance of species, directly impacted on how I had been feeling physically, emotionally and mentally.

This was just the beginning of my own health journey. It started up close and personal. That is why I constantly hear my patients say they feel like I really 'get' them. I've been there myself and continue to unravel the mystery day by day for my patients too.

I won't lie and say this was easy. My first thought after realizing what the results were telling me, was, *"Oh no, what can I now actually eat?"* It initially felt overwhelming.

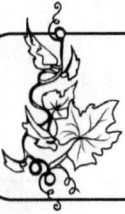

But, once I understood why food choices are so important, I started to look for alternatives and the health food store became my hunting ground.

The first three days were definitely the toughest. I had to focus on new supplements to take, foods to avoid and deal with strong cravings. Once I got through these initial days, I began to find a rhythm with the diet and supplements, and it became easier. I was still experiencing some gut symptoms for the first couple of weeks, but I'd been forewarned to hang in there and that things would gradually settle down.

By week three I experienced a big change, one that continues to convince me to this day of the success of this form of treatment. Twenty painful years of IBS gut symptoms had resolved.

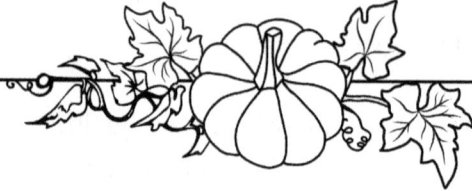

For the first time in two decades...

- my mind was clear

- my gut was functioning as it should

- my emotions were stable, and I was off the IBS emotional roller-coaster

- my poo was 10 out of 10

- I felt more than hope, I felt like I was back in control of my body and health

Since then, I have not looked back. I still need to tweak things here and there because I am human, and I fall off the wagon every now and then too. But doing the poo test and sorting out how to uniquely balance my microbiota was by far the most effective and life changing thing I have done for myself, my body and mind.

A clinical assessment tool that I use in clinic to understand a patient's gut function is the Rome IV criteria. This is a reasonably new (as of June 2016) set of criteria for diagnozing functional gastrointestinal (GI) disorders. It now reflects how functional bowel disorders are described and diagnozed. In particular these criteria help doctors, naturopaths and other health professionals to consistently categorize different types of IBS.

Irritable Bowel Syndrome (IBS)

There is a topic of conversation that is often repeated in my clinic. This is because the symptoms of IBS that relate to the Rome IV criteria fit a large number of people. Given that one in seven adults suffer from IBS it's a big part of my work in the gut health arena.

The prevalence of this non-pathological condition is now helped by the reclassification of symptoms and acknowledgement of the gut-brain connection. In fact, the updated Rome IV criteria now recognizes these symptoms:

- Motility disturbance (which can mean things moving too fast or too slow through the digestive system)
- Visceral hypersensitivity (commonly known as belly ache)
- Altered mucosal and immune function (inflammation and spasms)
- Altered gut microbiota (what this book is all about)
- Altered central nervous system processing (neurocognitive symptoms such as mind going blank, foggy brain, poor concentration and sleep disturbance)

Jessica's IBS Story

Jessica was 34 and presented with a typical IBS picture. Gut pain was a daily constant linked to everything she ate and every time she ate a meal. Her stool had changed – she had a need to rush to the toilet after every meal. This meant that she was IBS subtype D (D is for diarrhea.) There was a definite change in frequency. She had aches and pains, which affected her weight training and fitness at the gym, something she had been passionate about and loved.

So, like most of us, Jessica googled whatever she could find to help herself. If you've ever done this, one of the things you will likely come across is the fermentable oligosaccharides, disaccharides, monosaccharides and polyols (FODMAP) diet.

The FODMAP diet aims to restrict the consumption of fermentable foods to reduce IBS symptoms. FODMAPs are a group of sugars that are not completely digested as they travel through our digestive system. As FODMAPs pass into the large intestine these sugars ferment and produce gas, bloating/distention, wind and then a change in the function of the bowel.

Refer to the Appendix at the back of this book to familiarize yourself with a list of FODMAP containing vegetables.

The list of FODMAP foods is quite varied and simply by reducing your intake of these foods you can actually reduce the amount of fermentation in the gut. This will often reduce IBS symptoms – a great result for those wishing to address IBS. Once you try it with determination, you'll experience results firsthand, but the results can come at a hefty cost.

This is exactly what Jessica did, and because she was diligent, she got the results she desired. But it is hard to maintain the FODMAP diet and more importantly, in the longer term it simply does not address the key issue, which is the absence of certain gut bacteria. It targets symptoms without activating your own unique code.

For many people who try it, the results are good, but only last short term. So, despite sticking diligently to the diet, Jessica's symptoms returned even when she continued to restrict her diet to following FODMAP guidelines.

By the time Jessica got to me she had been on a highly restricted diet for over a year. She was now also highly stressed. Her stool sample revealed an undergrowth of key bacteria, and this was contributing to her symptoms. In the longer term if this was not addressed, it would have resulted in malabsorption and continued to impact her health, energy and mood too.

The key was to build the missing bacteria back up.

The purpose being to restore the diversity of bacteria present to enable Jessica to breakdown the full variety of fibers and sugars, including those that naturally contain FODMAPs.

The first signs we were on the right path was the reduction in pain and bloating. Jessica noticed further improvements with the firming-up of her stool and a reduction in the frequency of her bowel movements.

So far, so good. Maintaining Jessica's '10 out of 10 stool' was a key goal. The next thing was to very slowly build more diversity in Jessica's bacteria so that the strict diet restrictions were only a temporary part of her treatment. Finally, we worked on the importance of rotating the variety of foods that were previously problematic to being eaten once every four days.

Jessica was overjoyed to have her energy back, a clear mind, and no more foggy brain. Most importantly, those digestive symptoms that had consumed Jessica's attention every day, were absent, allowing her to focus on what really mattered: her life!

Deep down in the depths of an IBS sufferer is a sensitive soul trying to figure out their way in the world without being battered with symptoms all the time. These people tend to be givers and nurturers but often put themselves last on the list to receive. It's time to turn this around and give back some love and energy to your gut. It's time to nurture you.

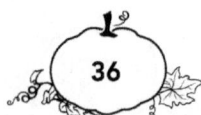

Sandy's Mood and Self-Harm Story

One of the first times the gut-brain connection really jumped out at me was early on in my career. A young teen, Sandy, came to see me.

Sandy's mother, Helena, had already been a patient and encouraged her daughter to get my help. For some time prior to our session, Sandy had become distant, avoidant and non-responsive to her family's attempts to help her. Helena subsequently found Sandy had been cutting herself. The situation was very complex for the family and everyone's stress levels were stretched to capacity.

I felt the weight of the situation and wanted to do whatever I could. I suggested a stool sample and testing of brain neurotransmitter function, but I was clear: where there was 'work' to be done, Sandy must agree and be the one to do it.

There is no point in doing all this investigative work and then not following through to address the results of testing. Expecting things to change without doing what it takes to change, is futile. I advised that Sandy needed to be on board too as there might be dietary changes and supplements to take and a few lifestyle tweaks.

Young girls go through such a challenging developmental shift between the ages of 13 and 17. So many things change for them at this age from puberty, identity, and sexuality. I am lucky I have some amazing people I work with, one of whom is a highly educated personal trainer who is a walking biochemistry encyclopedia. His special interest area is understanding the training needs of young teenage girls and what is happening to them biochemically at this age. He wrote me an email after a training session when we were trying to unravel the complexity of female teens. His email read:

"Hey Karls,

This is an awesome quote from Pipher's, Reviving Ophelia (p. 19). It underpins much of the reason behind my research choice, it embodies what happens to young girls as they transition from young girl to adolescent. Something dramatic happens to girls in early adolescence.

They crash and burn in a social developmental Bermuda Triangle. In early adolescence...they lose their resiliency and optimism and become less curious and inclined to take risks. They lose their assertive, energetic personalities and become more deferential, self-critical and depressed.

They report great unhappiness with their own bodies... boys are suffering too, make no mistake about it, but their dilemma is a different one from the girls, and their needs should be the subject of other research. Girls deserve our undivided attention; it is long overdue. As girls go through school, their self-esteem plummets, and the danger of depression increases."

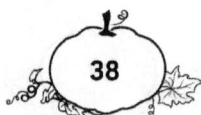

For Sandy, we could see this scenario playing out in real life. The key areas of change needing to be addressed were:

- Eating
- Sleep
- Exercise

Whatever habits a person has around these three areas of life will directly impact on their physical, emotional and mental health.

During Sandy's first consult with me she never made eye contact. Honestly, I didn't think I was going to get through to her at all. It didn't seem that she wished to engage with me. However, I received a telephone call from Helena after Sandy left.

Helena said, *"My daughter thinks you are kooky and she wants to work with you."* "Phew," I thought, *"no pressure, Karlene!"*

There is a duty of care to work with mental health conditions in collaboration with a care team of professionals and family who are involved in caring for the person. I take this duty of care very seriously and feel gratified to be considered a collaborator in each patient's medical care team. Sandy's team all wanted Sandy to get better and I felt that she was ready to step up and get better. So, in my role as a nutritionist and naturopath I stepped up and we did the stool test! Imagine the degree of difficulty in selling the idea of a poo test to a depressed and anxious teen!

We also did the neurotransmitter test and I put together a tough and personalized gut protocol that involved balancing the gut microbiota to ensure brain function was optimal.

I'd be lying if I said it was easy, however, the gut microbiota report confirmed that her gut imbalance had a significant impact on her mental health.

To activate her cure, Sandy would have to stop feeding the sugar-hungry bacteria. She needed to give up all sugar and fruit and improve her vegetable intake. First I had to convince her to do a poo test and then I had to tell her to stop eating sweets! Luckily, I believe in what I do and I knew that the changes in her gut would change her life!

Sandy also needed to take a specific probiotic to improve her GABA neurotransmitter production. (Gamma aminobutyric acid (GABA) is a naturally occurring amino acid that works as an inhibitory neurotransmitter in your brain. GABA produces a calming effect by inhibiting the brain's anxiety signals and settles your nervous system.

I also needed to supplement her diet to improve dopamine production. Initially, it was four weeks of intense work and remember, this work involved a care team helping Sandy with her emotional and psychological issues, so you must ensure that if you have mental health symptoms that you see yourself as requiring a holistic approach. By all means treat the gut, but ensure that your doctor, psychologist and family or friends are collaborating together for your treatment.

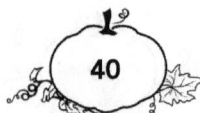

Sandy's neurotransmitter test results showed a significant lack of dopamine. This was interesting because most anti-depressants address serotonin but not dopamine. This meant I needed to also weave into Sandy's gut protocol the specific nutrients she required to assist in the production of this mood-elevating neurotransmitter. This is a prime example of when treatment protocols need to be super specific and personalized. There is never a generic, one size fits all solution.

What surprised me the most was the follow-up flow visit conducted at the four-week mark to see how things were going. Helena dropped Sandy to my clinic for the consult. She wanted her daughter to have private time with me without her presence. As I answered the door Sandy accidently dropped the pile of pathology reports she had been holding. She started laughing as we scrambled to pick up the papers. She laughed her way through our consult, her eyes bright and alive.

At the end when her mother picked her up, we waved goodbye. I remember watching the car drive away thinking, *"What the...?!!"* I called Helena a bit later to check in. *"Who was that?"* I asked. Helena replied, *"I know right? What a turnaround!"*

Later I asked Helena what she thought had been the key element that turned things around? *"It was the poo test,"* she said. We discussed the multi-factorial approach to address mental health which included psychology, counseling and behavioral therapy, anger and stress management as well as finding creative and physical outlets to direct energy and engage the mind. We also discussed how addressing gut health and digestion improved outcomes such as energy, focus, confidence and importantly, sleep.

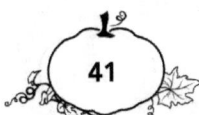

> If we treat the *whole* person, they get a whole lot better!

Sandy could so easily have balked at the poo test or stopping sweets but as they say in the classics, when the going gets tough, the tough get going and Sandy smashed it!

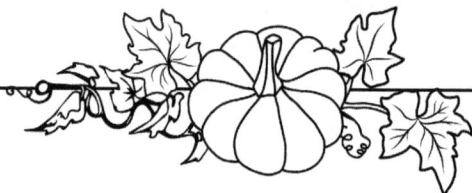

Mary's Sugar Addiction Story

When sugar-hungry gut bacteria have you in their grip, they will not let go easily or peacefully. We all know that too much sugar and processed food with hidden sugars is not good for us. In Damon Gameau's *That Sugar Film* he becomes the test subject and ends up with fatty liver from eating so called, *health foods, let alone sweets and treats!* Despite all the known benefits of quitting sugar, the reality is that quitting is not that simple.

Your sugar cravings are not a reflection of a 'sweet tooth' or poor will power, but sugar-specific bacteria demanding to be fed sugar. These bacteria gain a dominance in the gut that favors their own growth and suppresses the growth of other bacteria required for a healthy balance.

Mary's Sugar Addiction Story

This was the case for Mary who believed she had a huge 'sweet tooth.' She worked in a very high stress job and shared offices with people who all chased the 3pm sugar hit. Mary's job also included gifts of gratitude from patients and other staff members in the form of chocolate. Mary was very good at what she did, so the gifts were frequent. This was all too tempting for Mary's poor sugar-addicted gut.

Sadly, the race for the energy that Mary and her colleagues seeks can never be won. Sugar highs predict sugar lows that result in craving sugar once more. The sugar intake contributes to inflammation, acidity and, you guessed it, more fatigue. Every single drop of sucrose creates two molecules of D-Lactic acid. This takes the mitochondria inside your body extra adenosine triphosphate (ATP) cycles to break down. The ATP cycle simply refers to your body's process for making energy from the food you eat. The key message here is that your body has to work very hard to reverse the negative effects of eating sugar.

> *Eating sugar depletes your energy rather than giving you energy.*

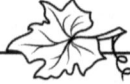

Mary habitually used sugar hits to counteract her afternoon slumps, headaches, brain fog and huge energy dropouts – unknowingly feeding the problem. On top of that she suffered insomnia and mild anxiety, compounding the sugar high-sugar low vicious cycle.

In the end the only way to treat this negative spiral is to cut the supply. Whether it be that you quit 'cold turkey' or through a slow weaning process – anticipate that your goal, once achieved, liberates you from the sugar rollercoaster. Mary didn't know how much the sugar had controlled her life until she gave it up. The aches and pains disappeared, her energy levels stabilized and improved, brain fog lifted, and her mental clarity returned. Not surprisingly, her anxiety and insomnia symptoms also improved.

What gut-healing requires from you

Fixing your gut microbial balance is not a quick easy fix. It takes an investment of your energy, time, money, focus and commitment. Change is a process, not a flick of the switch, so please do not doubt yourself if you succumb to cravings or relapse into old habits.

Lasting change is your goal, and quite often something important is learnt from a relapse. Please don't view a relapse as a negative

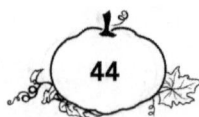

for your inner critic to scold you and leave you stuck in a sense of shame or helplessness. Instead see that food as having a quality that represents what's missing in your life.

- If it was ice-cream, perhaps see it as an instant gratification of a desire for sweetness.

- Now identify how that may be missing in your everyday experience of life.

- Next reflect on how you experienced sweetness as a child. Was it hugs, compliments, attention, play or nurturing?

- Furthermore, reflect on how your forebears found sweetness in their lives – especially in nature.

How long has it been since you held a newborn and smelt that sweet newborn smell? Or bottle-fed an orphaned lamb or listened to birdsong and lay on your back gazing at the clouds. Or a kiss. A sweet delicate kiss that falls upon you like cherry blossoms in spring? Get my sweet drift. Your apparent relapse is actually now a bridge to what your heart and soul needs from life. Do not let your inner critic undermine your journey to health. You really can do it. Remind yourself that every investment in gut health will pay off – it always does!

As mental clarity returns, patients tell me they feel so empowered and even a little *Teflon* coated and righteous ;-)

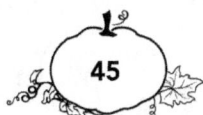

What's in the Bowl?

One of the key tasks along the way is, of course, to take a close look at what is in the toilet bowl. What is seen under the microscope is astounding. Through advanced testing and consultation, I offer an alternative path, providing hope for many conditions, especially those that have been labelled a 'syndrome' or a 'mystery', as well as those conditions that appear to be invisible, or labelled difficult to define. In the following chapters, you'll discover more about what to look for in the toilet bowl.

If you have ever been put in the 'too hard basket' or felt like you've tried *everything* to solve your biggest health mystery. If you haven't yet exhausted every option, and if you haven't had a professional poo sample test and analysis, then testing is essential so that you can address the cause, not just manage the symptoms.

The Sweet Spot

We are learning more and more about the gut, as research continues. What we already know is that we share a special symbiotic relationship with bacteria (and also viruses and fungi) and that there is a delicate balance.

The symbiotic nature of this relationship is important in health as it basically means 'living together for mutual benefit'. Achieving the balance of this mutual relationship is what I term, 'the sweet spot.'

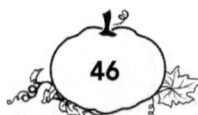

Our goal is to keep ourselves in the *sweet spot*.

A vast array of different species need to co-exist in the gut.

When in you're in the sweet spot, with everything in balance, they all contribute and work together to maintain homeostasis and great health.

Gut diversity - and balance - are two essential keys to your health and wellbeing.

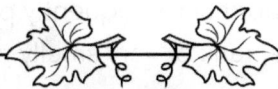

Chapter 1 - Take Home Highlights

FACT: A symbiotic relationship exists between each individual person and the bacteria, viruses and fungi which reside in their gut; where a healthy balance exists, we live with each other for mutual benefit.

- Metabolic acidosis often results from an imbalance in the types and numbers of bacteria present in the gut – symptoms can include headache, fatigue, weakness, nausea, vomiting, rapid heartbeat and long deep breaths

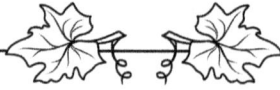

- Working with a practitioner and stool testing are important considerations for those who have a diagnozed medical condition, or unexplained symptoms of any kind

- Keep a chart of your symptoms and also a food diary – refer to the Appendix 1

- Start getting into the habit of looking at what's in the toilet bowl before you flush it away every day

- It is not normal to frequently produce stinky, offensive, rank or very smelly poos

- Check in on how you are feeling after you have eaten

- Notice the foods that you crave and foods you avoid

- Commit for the long haul – change requires your energy, time, money, focus and commitment – it's not about managing the symptoms – it is about addressing the cause to prevent the symptoms and create wellbeing!

BIGGEST HEALTH MYSTERIES SOLVED

INVISIBLE DISEASES

Revealing things that cant be seen

The only thing invisible about so-called, 'invisible diseases', is that we can't always see physical evidence.

Invisible diseases are conditions such as arthritis, diabetes, chronic fatigue syndrome, fibromyalgia, many other autoimmune conditions, as well as mental illnesses. Quite often people living with 'invisible illness' feel criticized and misunderstood. This commonly fuels frustration at the lack of understanding from others or hopelessness directed at themselves and their symptoms.

Living with an invisible disease is often about surviving not thriving. Getting through today becomes the focus and when a symptom becomes aggravated, it can be a minute-by-minute energy vacuum.

Complex and chronic health conditions often present with symptoms that don't make sense when looked at individually, however when I step back, it's clear that the body is just trying to maintain homeostasis and heal itself.

The body is constantly providing signs. In my work, I am looking for that common thread that links them all together. Often when I take a new case history, people will say, *"I don't know if this is related…but I also get blah blah."* I say YES of course it is related because it is within YOU, all these things are related…and then we go back to the gut.

- Allergies and food intolerances
- Arthritis, especially rheumatoid

- Cancer
- Chronic fatigue syndrome
- Fibromyalgia
- Depression and mental Illness
- Diabetes
- Digestive disorders such as coeliac, colitis and IBS
- Migraine and headache
- Heart conditions
- Lupus
- Lyme disease
- Multiple sclerosis
- Infertility
- Sjogren's syndrome

These are some names of the many invisible illnesses we know. Bacteria, viruses and fungi are also invisible, but they occupy a crucial role in our health and our body's homeostasis. For example, most of us live in modern, sterile homes and workplaces and our internal digestive system reflects this modern reduction in microbial diversity and unfortunately, it does not promote good health.

The rise of sterile home environments appears to be progress but it's associated decline of microbial diversity has been inextricably linked to chronic health problems and the increase of 'invisible illnesses.'

Imagine there is an invisible factory going on inside you controlled by bacteria, viruses and fungi.

- These can be good bosses in the factory making the factory work well to create great gut health or

- bad bosses, causing troubling symptoms.

The question for you is: is your home environment working for or against you in maintaining your health and wellbeing?

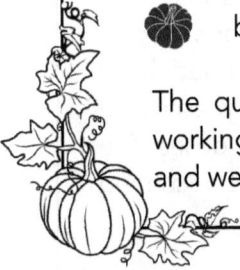

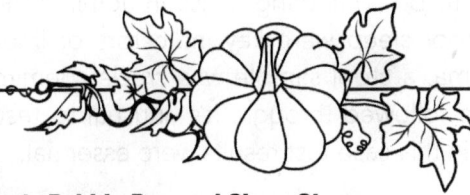

Baby Jemima's Pebble Poo and Sleep Story

Beautiful eight-month-old Jemima and her mother visited me in clinic. Jemima's mother was worried because Jemima was terribly constipated. Jemima only passed a little pebble-poo every few days, always with great pain and difficulty, despite being breastfed and eating really simple and clean foods.

The other main issue was Jemima's sleep. My goodness how did this baby operate with such a small amount of sleep? Jemima would go down for 20 minutes at best during the day, and only sleep for two hours maximum at any one time during the night.

Baby Jemima's Pebble Poo and Sleep Story

Jemima's mother was exhausted and at her wits end. She had tried everything including laxatives suitable for an eight-month-old. Probiotics had also been recommended by a health professional, and the doctor continued prescribing various laxatives, but Jemima kept needing higher doses. The problem was not being solved and her mother was becoming more anxious and exhausted by the day.

There had to be something amiss in Jemima's little gut, as poo and poor sleep were key indicators of imbalance. For baby Jemima, a stool sample was crucial. Jemima's mother agreed and followed through. It's unusual to test a baby so young but in this case test results were essential.

The test results were clear: Jemima's challenge was mainly about microbiota *overgrowth*, including the probiotics being administered. These probiotics had exacerbated the overgrowth and were only adding to the problem. This included *Bifidobacterium*, which is beneficial in the right amounts, however, when in overgrowth it can cause constipation.

Once we addressed the bacterial overgrowth, the results were phenomenal. As evidenced by the many photos Jemima's mother proudly sent me, Jemima went from pooing pebbles that were very difficult to pass, to the most magnificent poos ever. Jemima was a happy baby, but until we addressed the gut imbalance, Jemima's symptoms were telling us things were not so happy on the inside.

The way we develop our microbiota in our gut from birth is an area of research that is constantly evolving. There is a current indication that the preborn baby has quite a sterile environment in the gut containing little to no bacteria and that the first inoculation of microbiota comes during vaginal delivery at birth. It is then followed by further inoculation by breastfeeding. Further research indicates the first inoculation comes from the mother's own microbiome.

The way commensal (symbiotic) bacteria colonize in the gut of a newborn follows a particular pattern. Caesarean birth, lack of breastfeeding and or possibility of antibiotics (taken by the mother pre-birth or delivery) will all impact the development of the baby's gut microbiota.

The prolonged use of probiotics and/or laxatives will also influence the growth of certain bacteria. In my experience, these interventions can contribute to overgrowth when used incorrectly. Remember it is important to always aim for the homeostasis sweet-spot for everything and everyone.

In babies I am particularly interested in:

- Poo
- Sleep
- Skin

Symptoms across these areas can often be attributed to microbiota imbalance and overgrowth and can be so easily fixed by restoring your baby's natural balance.

Scoring your poo!

I always ask my patients to give me a report on their poo. *"Give me a score out of 10 for your poo,"* I say. I know perfection doesn't exist. But when it comes to poo this is where I strive for the perfect '10 out of 10.'

I am forever referring to what is in the toilet bowl, and it astounds me that so many people don't know or are too embarrassed to look! As young children we had no problem talking about poo, but somewhere along the line we were conditioned to stop that conversation. Isn't it ironic though, that the jokes people laugh at the most are right back there, in the toilet! Take it from me, checking in on your poo is an important health check that you can perform daily.

Two of the most used tools in my clinic are the *Bristol Stool Chart and my Mood Poo Chart*. I am always at the ready when patients tell me that their stool is "normal". They are often surprised to see so many variations regarding what is "normal" right in front of them. I see them go into deep thought as they ponder their poo. What was it today?

Personality and Mood Poo Chart

I believe that understanding our poo is so important, that I have taken the original concept of the original Bristol Stool Chart to the next level.

I developed my own stool chart that also considers understanding your poo's 'personality'. Yes, different poo types suggest different moods and health symptoms. I give the different types of poo personalities that are easily remembered and represent the different variations.

Remember we are always looking for the sweet spot and that starts with the perfect 10 out of 10 poo.

The answer to life, the universe and everything

Just in case you were wondering the answer to life, the universe, and everything…is not 42. According to me, it's just four! Four is the number of the perfect poo on the **Bristol stool chart** and my *Personality and Mood Poo Chart.*

Poo Number Four is:

- Smooth like a sausage, not dry or cracked.
- It maintains its form when it hits the water.
- It is easy to pass.
- There is a sense of complete emptying.
- And finally, it sinks, it does not float!

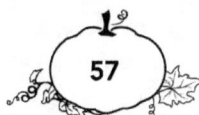

ORIGINAL BRISTOL STOOL CHART

KARLENE'S STOOL CHART PERSONALITY PROFILE
For Optimal Mood And Health

WHAT TO DO TO GET TO THE PERFECT #4 POO
Mr and Mrs Smooth

TYPE 1
Hard Lumps

Mr Pebble Pants
He feels like he's stressed and under pressure. Life seems like a real squeeze. He's dry, dehydrated, a little on the scarce side, and hard to pass.

Drink more water, remember he needs hydration. Add psyllium husks to your breakfast or salads. Add magnesium and more vegetable fibers. Alkalize.*

TYPE 2
Sausage shape but lumpy

Mrs Cranky Pants
She's irritable and difficult to please. She almost looks like a sausage, but has more volume and feels better with more hydration.

She needs more vegetable fibres and lets get hydrated. Alkalize.*

TYPE 3
Sausage with cracks

Mr Kransky Pants
His mood indicates some cracks are showing, just like the cracks on the hard sausage that he forms. His goal is to become smoother, softer, more gentle and easy to pass.

Add more vegetable fibers

TYPE 4
Smooth and soft like a sausage. Easy to pass

Mr & Mrs Smooth Pants
These smooth operators have found the sweet spot! They confidently get things done and are smooth to all things means they are a pleasure to pass. Mr and Mrs Smooth indicate balance inside you and in your health and mood too.

BLISS

TYPE 5
Blobs with clear edges

Mrs Blobby Pants
She's lost her personality, and lacks structure. She feels lost and a little fluffy about life.

Needs bone broth*

MR & MRS SMOOTH'S GOLDEN RULES
1. Drink more water
2. Eat more vegetable fibers
3. Try bone broth
4. Alkalize

TYPE 6
Fluffy with ragged edges

Mr Fluffy Pants
He's avoiding everything. He's anxious and squishy, scared and thinks it's not fair.

Needs bone broth and more soluble and insoluble vegetable fibres*

TYPE 7
Liquid

Mrs Squirty Pants
Oh dear! She can't leave the house and doesn't know what to eat. Confused and worried.

Needs bone broth, more soluble and insoluble vegetable fibres. 3-5 days only, slippery elm and charcoal.*

Copyright Karlene Georgiadis 2022 www.karlenegeorgiadis.com.au

*seek medical advice if symptoms persist.

What your poo 'looks' like does surprisingly reflect on your external mood not just your internal gut health. The tiny microbiota living within us, are working with and for us or working against us. They affect the way we look on the outside and how we feel on the inside.

We initially inherit our microbiota from our mothers and as we grow up, our diet, lifestyle and the environment we in live greatly shape our microbiome.

As mentioned earlier, a dysfunctional microbiome has now been linked to many of the invisible health issues we've discussed so far. Even autism, cancer, obesity, severe allergies, psoriasis, acne, eczema, asthma, anxiety, depression and more have been linked to the balance in our gut.

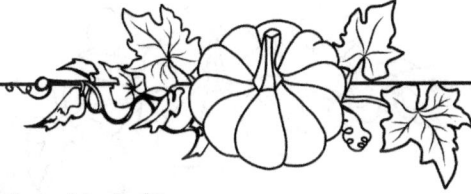

Monica's Endometriosis Story

Monica had a long history of menstrual irregularities that finally landed her with the diagnosis of endometriosis. Arriving at a diagnosis was a long and arduous twisting path of many visits to doctors and specialists. There were many blood tests, scopes, ultrasounds and a laparoscopy.

"Endo" is another one of those invisible diseases. This is where endometrial tissue that grows and sheds from the uterus each month, can grow in other areas of the body. The uterus is hormonally activated, it sheds and bleeds and can cause severe pain and irritation to the organs where the tissue grows. Approximately 11% of women are affected by endometriosis.

While it is not regarded as an autoimmune condition, endometriosis classification is currently under review. It is certainly connected to the immune system with inflammation and pain being key factors associated with immune responses. These can increase the risk of concurrent autoimmune conditions and the risk of vaginal infection, as well as chronic endometritis and pelvic inflammatory disease.

This was the case for Monica.

Monica's symptoms included heavy and painful periods with massive energy drops that left her pale and shaking, as well as consistently low iron and regular bacterial infection, mainly bacterial vaginosis. Her treatment involved multiple rounds of antibiotics and weeks of pain killers. The reality was that there were approximately only five days each month where Monica had no symptoms. She felt trapped on a horror rollercoaster of pain, despair and confusion.

For some time, Monica came to see me to help manage the symptoms, but despite my recommendation of a stool test, she didn't want to do the test. So we focused on hormones and nutrients which gave some relief, but I finally convinced Monica that we'd never resolve this without a stool sample.

As usual, the stool report was the vital piece of the puzzle we needed to further improve Monica's hormonal profile as well as address bacterial overgrowth that was feeding the bacterial vaginosis (BV). Monica had to dig deep and stop feeding the bacteria with sugar. We rectified the imbalance by alkalizing and using bone broth and loads of vegetables (as listed in Chapter 5 including soluble and insoluble vegetables)

The best part of this story is that Monica is most firmly now in the driver's seat of her health. She has claimed back her vitality and is thriving. She knows what to do and when to reign in her diet to feed the right bacteria well. She also knows when she needs to rest and when to push through. Monica monitors her need for pain killers and is aware of when she can do other things to help. Most importantly she knows when she needs to go to hospital, which these days is rarely at all.

It is important to note that gut health is intricately connected to hormonal and menstrual health. Not only do they share the same space in the pelvic cavity but also pain, spasms and contractions in one directly affect the other. Sometimes, it is hard to differentiate where the pain stems from. Addressing gut health and microbiota has a massive positive impact on hormonal health, as well as addressing bacterial overgrowths that can impair reproductive health.

Everyone has a unique microbiota pattern, the natural mix of bacteria found in the gut. The microbiota co-evolved with us and live with us in a symbiotic relationship as human health is closely linked to this microbiota. The diversity and make up of our microbiome is influenced by factors such as diet, genetics, age, ethnicity, medications and supplements, lifestyle, environment and stress levels.

It's interesting to think that your physical environment – where you live, work and play – affects your gut health so closely too. The situations you choose to put yourself in have a large impact on your internal health. Research even shows that owning a family pet will affect your microbiota, in fact, pets will often share a similar make up of organisms to people in the household. You are unique, your story, your environment, your background, what you eat and how you do almost everything is unique to you. Therefore, your microbiota is unique and has its own story too.

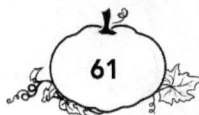

You can add indoor plants, pets and walks in nature to enrich your microbiota input.

> "I learnt so much about gut health from doing the test. Until you get a clear picture of the state of your individual microbiome you really are just stabbing in the dark with trying to find solutions. I didn't realize how many of my symptoms were related to my gut. Lower back pain, mental fog and forgetfulness, poor sleep, lethargy etc. After having the test, it did give me more motivation to commit to the protocol, as I felt that what I was doing was customized for my circumstances rather than a generic program. Somehow it made it seem more worth sticking to"
>
> - Emma, from Jan Juc, Victoria, Australia

Animals and Poo

Even the digestive symptoms of other mammals provides the key to help understand the health of that animal better.

One of my pastimes is to hang out on a farm where my daughter rides horses. I am not much into riding horses myself, so my daughter is my hero in this arena. However, I am fascinated by horse poo. Go figure – at this stage of the book, you're probably not surprised. Shovelling shit is a helpful thing to do on a farm but

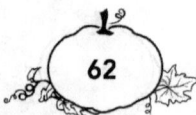

just as it is with humans, you can also tell the health of an animal by observing their excrement. Some horses are fed so well that their poo gets eaten by birds.

Horses, like humans, rely on fiber in their diet to feed their microbiota. It is interesting to note that horses can't vomit, so if they eat the wrong things, it's detrimental to their health. Colic for a horse is very serious.

I recall picking up poo in a horse paddock one day and remarking on the dark colour. The horse was big, yet the nuggets of poo he produced were small and looked quite dry. I am not a vet, but I knew the poo didn't look right. I discussed this with the horse's owner and suggested she get the horse checked by a vet. Later I learnt that the horse had a stomach ulcer. It was treated and the horse recovered.

> When I observe poo, whether it is horse or human, I can recognize when something is off balance. Quite often, simple and easy steps can be immediately taken to rectify the problems.

Healthy balance is always the key, which is why it is important to not over do any one thing. It is unwise to go down the rabbit hole of following a diet that concentrates on cutting out food groups or even overconsuming specific food types. Everything has its rightful place; the place is called the land of 'balance.'

Chapter 2 -Take Home Highlights

FACT: The only thing that is invisible about invisible diseases, is that we can't always see physical evidence of the disease.

- Just because you can't see the disease, this doesn't mean no disease exists.

- Invisible diseases can be just as physically, emotionally and mentally. exhausting as conditions where there is physical evidence of disease.

- The time for conventional medicine to better understand invisible diseases is now.

- Switch your mindset over from surviving to thriving – starting today!

- Start by getting curious about your diagnosis – all your symptoms are related.

- Next, get curious about your poo – what does it look like and smell like?

- Know your shit – refer to my Mood and Poo Chart – give your shit a rating every day.

Get to know the stool chart and aim for number four, which is smooth like a sausage and not dry or cracked, it holds its form when it hits the water, it is easy to pass, there is a sense of complete emptying and it does not float, it sinks.

Remember: Balance is the goal and balance is the way!

Chapter Three

EXPOSING MYTHS

IT'S ALL ABOUT BALANCE

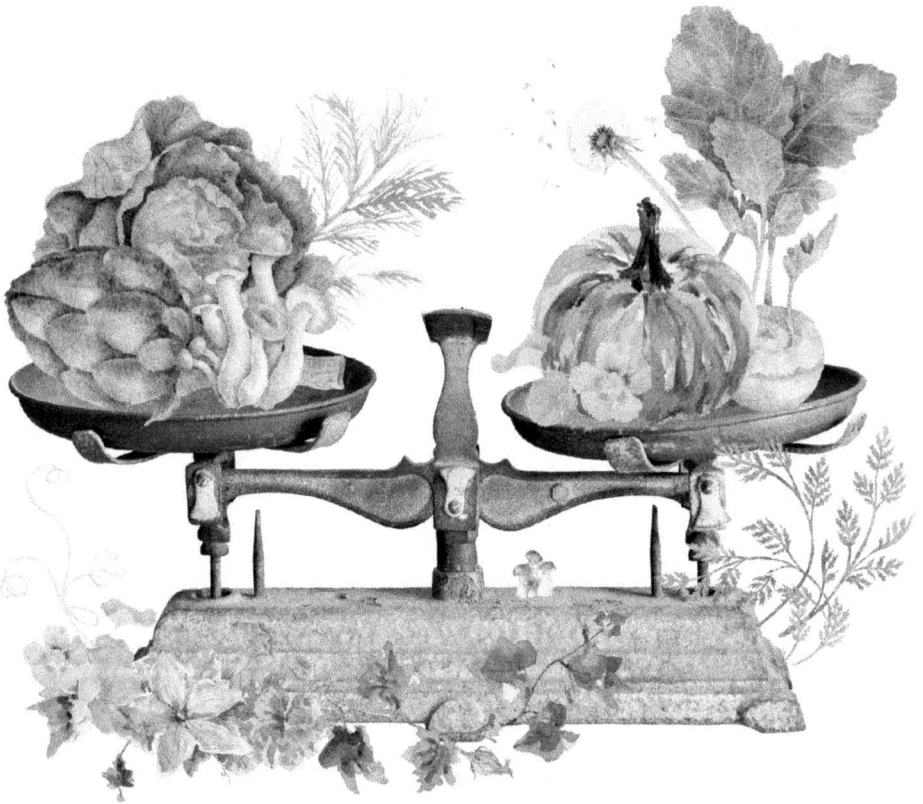

*Exposing the myths in Gut Health to Find
the Sweet Spot. Everything is dose dependent*

There is no such thing as 'good' and 'bad' bacteria. All bacteria should be there, in fact, the greater the diversity, the better.

The question that arises is, what is that balance, how many of each type of bacterium should there be?

There is an optimal number and if you have one type of bacterium in overgrowth, there will be another type in undergrowth.

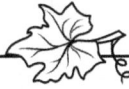

Imagine an old-fashioned set of scales. Too much weight on one side leads to an imbalance and the scales swing out of balance into a precarious state of imbalance. This is a helpful way to think about your gut bacteria in the event of ill health, but a healthy balance is achievable.

It is about jiggling the numbers and making a dietary or medicinal correction; an excess requires suppression. This might mean using an anti-microbial herb, but also at the same time, it would require that you stop consuming whatever it is that has been feeding them. That means a change in diet.

On the other side you need to be mindful of building up what is needed to fill the gap created with the suppression. It's not just about adding more fiber, you also need the right balance of bacteria that will break down the fiber.

What comes first, fiber or the bacteria?

The answer is the bacteria, and the next step is to feed the bacteria the *right* fibers.

I am not a big fan of excess or unwarranted fermented foods, such as the latest fads like kombucha and kefir or sauerkraut. I use these things sparingly and with respect because they are powerful foods that can overgrow specific bacteria and inadvertently contribute to a highly acidic system, creating an allergy scenario.

> Everything is dose-dependent.
> Everything has a sweet spot.

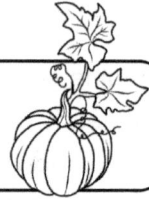

This is so important in terms of gut bacteria and in the arena of endocrinology.

Endocrinology

Endocrinology is the study of the hormonal system in the human body, the system of glands that secrete active hormones. Hormones are chemicals which affect the actions of different organ systems in the body. Hormones are communication messengers. Examples include thyroid hormone, growth hormone, and insulin.

The complexity of the hormonal system in relation to the immune system and how the body can turn on itself in autoimmunity is detailed and complex. I love treating complex cases, undoing the triggers for autoimmunity.

Hashimoto's is one of the many complex autoimmune conditions that I love to address via the gut.

I see complex cases like a giant jigsaw puzzle. As I put all the pieces together, the true picture comes into focus. I can help people really understand how they trigger their autoimmunity via the gut.

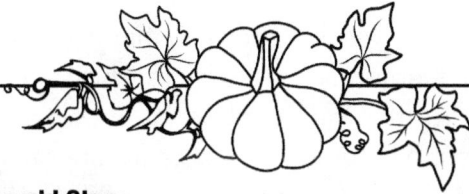

Jennie's Thyroid Story

Jennie was suffering terribly with autoimmune challenges. Her concerns started with Graves' disease, an overactive thyroid autoimmune condition. After treatment by her medical team, her thyroid then became underactive and she was diagnosed with Hashimoto's, an underactive autoimmune thyroid condition. She felt like she was bouncing all over the place. The task was to stabilize the condition in her digestive system, which meant supporting the pathways to regulation.

Jennie's worst symptoms of Hashimoto's were ongoing fatigue, a foggy brain and difficulty sleeping, making it so hard to be the mum she needed to be for her active young son and to work part-time.

Optimizing thyroid function requires a holistic approach. I first addressed her nutrient status, including iron and zinc, and rebalanced her gut health with a thorough protocol, and she unlocked her energy.

Making sure all of these things are present in the form of nutrient supply is key. This is followed by stabilizing the immune system. Everybody is different. Even if they have been diagnosed with the same condition. This is why I love poo-testing because it is so specific.

Jennie's stool test results showed that the balance of her microbiota was feeding an acid pattern which was presenting as fatigue. Added to this, her numbers of Eubacterium were zero. This can play out over time for people as a hormonal imbalance and this is exactly what was happening for Jennie. Her upper digestive symptoms also indicated she had gastro-esophageal reflux disease (GERD).

GERD/GORD

GERD is a very uncomfortable digestive disorder that occurs when acidic stomach juices, or food and fluids, back up from the stomach into the esophagus. GERD affects people of all ages, from infants to older adults.

For Jennie, these symptoms indicated the higher acid levels in her digestive system due to the overgrowth of lactic acid producing bacteria. This also provided a key sign that things were out of balance.

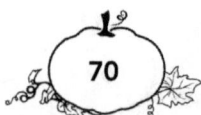

Being aware of this has allowed her to manage her symptoms and understand how the Hashimoto's was being triggered. She still needs to manage her medications and supplements, but once Jennie's days shifted from being "no energy, no joy" to days with "good energy levels", she reported seeing a "better future ahead."

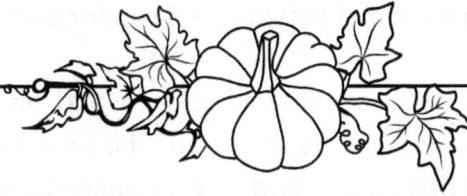

James' Sexual Dysfunction and Loss of Libido Story

If I was to list the most common challenges both men and women of all ages acknowledge when talking about their overall health, those topics would be:

1. Sleep
2. Loss of libido
3. Sexual dysfunction and
4. Infertility

Loss of libido can happen to anyone at any age regardless of gender. It should come as no surprise to learn that when your gut health function is optimal, then factors like hormonal balance, nutrient status and stress resilience all function optimally too. Liver function is also very much a part of this picture.

This is the picture that presented to me when James walked through my door. While only a young man in his early 40s, James had suffered low libido since his 20s.

Genetics and life's stresses were adding to his burden, however, once James completed a stool test, we identified the gut-causes of a frustrating issue that had plagued him for over two decades.

We corrected his microbiota imbalance and his gut function and absorption of nutrients improved. This lowered his need for ongoing supplementation, and he experienced the physical and sexual energy of his teen years.

While his wife was happy to have her passionate lover back again it's not just about sex. Expressing his love and affection physically via sex was not something James could substitute through buying gifts or flowers. This issue affected his self-esteem and sense of masculinity. He simply wanted to feel capable of being a good lover to his wife.

For so many of my patients, the cost of poor health is not just in the form of discomfort or fatigue, but it harms their sense of self-confidence and self-worth as they find themselves unable to live a healthy and normal life.

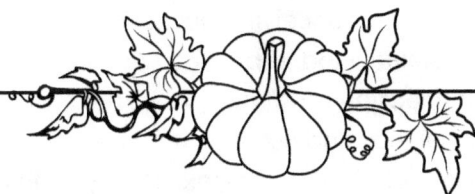

Lily's Infertility Story

Infertility, from a female perspective, is fraught with high emotions. Having studied a specialized fertility course only months after graduating as a naturopath back in 1998, I have a lot of experience addressing infertility and supporting women to improve their fertility both naturally and using in vitro fertilization (IVF).

Lily was in her late 30s. She was on an emotional rollercoaster journey of infertility and addressing this with IVF treatment. Each month Lily's hopes and expectations would build, only to be let down with the first show of blood. *"It is so emotionally draining,"* she admitted when I first saw her.

You might well assume that conception is confined to treatments that target the sexual and reproductive systems. I cannot emphasise enough that our sexual health is not somehow separate from our overall health. Everything and everyone is interconnected. I am fortunate to work in a collaborative way with some amazing practitioners and we each play complementary roles that translate into effective health outcomes.

If you have had difficulty conceiving but have only had interventions that target the sexual and reproductive systems, then please consider that conception is not just about the sperm fertilizing an egg. Hormonal balance and nutrient status rely heavily on gut and liver function, both obviously non-sexual players in conception. It also helps to put in place ways to regularly de-stress.

Imagine that a car is at a traffic light, stopped and waiting for the red light to turn to green. Imagine that the lights change but instead of there being a green light down the bottom, it is another red. It doesn't matter how fast the car is, or how experienced and skillful the driver is, if the light is still red. The light needs to be the right color before it is possible for the conception journey to continue.

Instead of being self-critical of yourself or your partner, I say let's optimize all your interconnected health systems to create a 'green light' for conception and pregnancy. The journey to conception can be such a private experience of monthly heartbreak that is invisible to family, friends and colleagues. Please practice self-care and compassion and seek professional support if your mindset shifts from feeling defeated to depressed.

Alongside genetic testing and all the biochemistry checks, the stool sample was the best way to ensure we had ticked every box to unravel Lily's mystery.

The steps we took were not only a great detox and reset for her, but also ensured the best possible nutrient status and a healthy bacterial profile. This profile is exactly what you pass to your newborn, through the vagina at birth. In caesarean birth, it is still

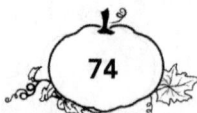

possible for a mother to gently transfer healthy bacteria from her vaginal flora to her newborn. Developing the baby's microbiota which then continues through feeding with the bacterial building properties of breast milk.

Lily's first pregnancy with IVF was successful and her story ended in one of life's greatest joys: giving birth to a healthy baby boy!

Her baby number two is on its way at the time of writing this book, but guess what's different about this pregnancy? Her second baby was conceived naturally, no intervention required!

Natalie's Polycystic Ovarian Syndrome (PCOS) Story

Polycystic ovarian syndrome (PCOS) isn't always easily identified. It's one of those challenges that can be tricky to treat.

If you spend any time with Dr Google you will find a general outline of the most common symptoms with a typical picture of this condition. But PCOS can have great variation in its blend of symptoms, reflecting the unique characteristics of its sufferers. We're all different. Not one of us is exactly the same. Once again, please avoid judging yourself if you don't fit the generic model of symptoms.

Conditions may present in obscure ways. PCOS symptoms can also morph over time, making PCOS harder to identify and track in some people. All hormonal imbalance conditions such as, PCOS require patient and thorough understanding. Usually, I do a lot of digging to identify the PCOS, except that it can be a moving target, with new or changing characteristics.

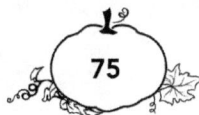

This is why I like to work with a team of health professionals. Sometimes that can include a doctor, endocrinology specialist, gastroenterologists, physiotherapist, chiropractor, osteopath, kinesiologist, hypnotherapist, the list continues. It is a team effort; each player has their niche role that combine so that you have every chance to thrive.

The prevalence of PCOS is as high as 26% in women of reproductive age. Primary characteristics of PCOS can include hyperandrogenism, anovulation, insulin resistance and neuroendocrine disruption. This syndrome features cysts which form on the ovaries, but this is not the cause of the disorder.

Some of the signs may include:

- No menstrual periods, or very irregular periods
- Excess body or facial hair
- Acne
- Pelvic pain
- Infertility
- Type 2 diabetes
- Obesity
- Obstructive sleep apnoea
- Mood disorders

So, it was a shock to me when Natalie walked into my clinic with none of these symptoms, however, she had been previously diagnosed with PCOS.

Natalie didn't come to see me for help with the PCOS diagnosis. She presented with a strange and extreme allergic reaction that covered her body in welts.

It's important to consider what the signs and symptoms are pointing towards, whilst also investigating hormones, the menstrual cycle and blood sugar regulation. In fact, many improvements can be made when a treatment supports hormones to be well-regulated. But this approach to treatment made no difference at all to the main issue Natalie was presenting with, so don't despair if you suffer PCOS but haven't yet responded to treatments. Natalie's allergic reactions came out of the blue and seemed to have no relation to diet, or to her external environment.

So instead of continuing to investigate where everyone else was looking, I went to where most don't look – yep, you guessed it - a stool sample.

Thank goodness that I did as the most unlikely bacteria showed up in the results. This included a few new ones, that after all my years of working in this field, some I had never even heard of before!

The protocol required for Natalie was the most unusual one I've created to date. This was one of those instances when I felt I was reading the tea leaves! I put each protocol together based on the evidence presented to me by the test result. Natalie's protocol was no exception. The complicating aspect in Natalie's case was the amine response that looked very much like histamines. Upon further investigation however, the picture revealed other amines that were being produced by the gut bacteria.

Reducing these was the key to decreasing Natalie's allergic response. Happily, it also had the result of regulating Natalie's hormones and balancing her blood sugar as well.

For the first time ever, Natalie began to get a regular period. She lost 12 kilograms and reduced her allergic reaction to zero: No more welts!. Now she knows her triggers, she keeps her gut bacteria balanced, and she happily reports her allergic reactions and the PCOS are completely under control!

These symptoms are a reminder of how your body is talking to you all the time. What is important, is that you recognize symptoms as signs of a need for a gut-correction. Once the cause is identified and the correction is translated into your tailored health and wellbeing protocol, it's simply a matter of doing what needs to be done to achieve great health.

If we don't initially listen to our body, symptoms can worsen and sometimes it's a dramatic wakeup call perhaps an emergency trip to the hospital, or sometimes it is the small accumulative symptoms that accrue overtime and one day you just can't get out of bed.

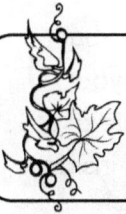

> Listen to all the ways that your body speaks to you through symptoms…and observe the quality of your poo.

Take a peek every day and check your number twos. Is your poo a number four? That's our goal!

Your relationship with your gut shapes how you feel about yourself moment to moment. It is often the thing that can drive a client to my door to seek help. But if you are reading this book, you are already doing something about it, so congratulations. As you read, remember to take lots of notes while you reflect on your life, physiology and health needs.

In the next chapter we'll take a peek at more symptoms and my straightforward solutions, but first let's check our Chapter Three highlights as shown below:

Chapter 3 - Take Home Highlights

FACT: Loss of libido and sexual dysfunction can happen to anyone at any age regardless of gender.

- There is a connection between optimal gut health function and optimal health across other body systems including hormonal system balance.

- Your age and the genes you inherit from your parents do not automatically determine your health – GERD/GORD is just one example of a condition where the health and function inside your gut plays a very important role too!

- There is also a connection between your liver function and both your hormonal balance and nutrient status.

- Your gut bacteria exert a big influence on the nutrients your body is able to absorb.

- A variety of bacteria are meant to be present in your gut and in the right balance.

- Addressing gut function involves looking for the upstream factors that cause your symptoms – I call this treating the root cause.

- Optimal gut function can mean the difference between requiring the assistance of IVF and not requiring the assistance of IVF to conceive.

- There is also a connection between optimal gut function and weight gain, or weight loss.

SYMPTOMS AND SOLUTIONS

YOU ARE YOUR MEDICINE

This is about the chemistry of the kitchen and the alchemy of the medicine within.

Your symptom picture is your unique message from your body. That picture is trying to tell you to take notice.

Helene's Parkinson's Story

Helene had fairly early stages Parkinson's Disease. Our consult was exhausting for her because staying still was quite a challenge. Her husband was also very unwell at the time, so it was a stretch for Helene to take the time out for herself. In fact, the time away from her husband caused her a lot of stress.

Like most people when they first receive a diagnosis, Helene had done a ton of research. She was in the hands of a good physician and specialist, yet she felt there might be more she could do. Her research led her to believe she would benefit from vegetarianism which involved her eating loads of vegetables and carbohydrates.

During our first consult I discovered Helene was crazy about golf! So how cruel for her that the Parkinson's symptoms meant she could no longer play her beloved golf! Helene was understandably devastated.

At this point I just had to convince Helene to do a stool test. Parkinson's is an autoimmune condition, and credible research shows that these conditions start in the gut.

What Helen's stool report showed was confronting because of how bad things were. The results were also exciting because it means that there was a lot that could be done! Helene's lack of diversity in her gut was alarming, it was almost sterile. Her poo was deficient in *all* types of bacteria. She didn't have one single overgrowth, which is extremely uncommon.

> I formulated a plan to build up all her bacteria again, much like a horticulturalist nurturing a barren landscape back to a thriving ecology.

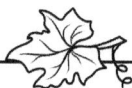

Contrary to her strict vegetarian diet, meat (as well as bone broth) returned to the family menu, which pleased her hubby and also started the healing process. I have been using and recommending bone broth for decades and it is finally being recognized for its benefits to the gut!

As this wonderfully determined woman embraced her new diet rich in bone broth, a wide variety of vegetables and meat, her gut microbiota began to flourish, and her health quickly improved.

Most importantly, within six weeks Helene was back on the golf course taking on nine holes and building herself up to18 holes. Whilst I'm passionate about health, it's when a patient can regain their quality of life, that my work is most rewarding!

Helene's specialist's words were, *"You don't look like you have Parkinson's anymore."* She later told me that members of her family regularly said, *"Whatever you are doing, don't stop."* Let's take a moment and reflect on how it all works.

A word on vegetarianism and vegan diets

As you may have gathered I am a big believer in meeting people where they are at. I work with test results and evidence-based recommendations. It is not my intention to get everyone eating meat nor is it to place anyone in an ethical dilemma based on their choices. Don't abandon your principles. I am here to make the best recommendations for you and your gut.

Being mostly plant based is part of that as this is where the wonderful fibres are in our food. However, there are times that the human gut needs some animal products to help restore balance and in these cases I ask for return to health to be the top priority. Consideration for achieving the best health outcomes as well as making the most ethical decisions, is what enables us to remain in balance and harmony with all living things.

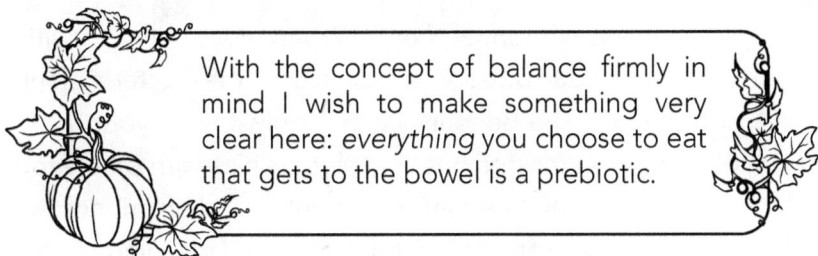

With the concept of balance firmly in mind I wish to make something very clear here: *everything* you choose to eat that gets to the bowel is a prebiotic.

By the time your food gets to your bowel, it is not just about feeding a 'poo making factory'. Absorption of nutrients for energy occurs further up the digestive tract, however, it is not all over by the time the fibers (the part that cannot be digested and absorbed) get to the large bowel. It is there that the mystery is revealed.

While Hippocrates said, *"All disease begins in the gut,* his wisdom can be extended to include: *"You are what your gut microbes metabolize (from) what you eat..."* and...before *maintaining a species-rich gut ecosystem through diet is a science-backed way to achieve a healthier lifestyle."* - Weizmann

It is these fibers that feed the bacteria, and the bacteria in turn have a process of producing each metabolite. These metabolites feed the colonocytes and what is required for the body to produce a myriad of nutrients. I am referring to nutrients such as folate, coenzyme Q10, tryptophan, tyrosine, vitamin K2 and more.

This then feeds your energy, your capacity to heal, your immune system, your brain function and capacity to think clearly, your mood, your sleep, and your hormonal system. This is the big picture of your life!

Can you see the potential here? When you get a healthy relationship with your gut and a balance of the bacteria doing great work for you, the benefits will not only flow to your health and vitality, it translates into healthy relationships with others too. Whether it be your intimate partner, parents, children, friends and colleges it all helps to create a rich fulfilling and meaningful life.

It all depends on whether you actually HAVE the bacteria that are required to do this important job. Next, it depends on whether you are actually feeding these bacteria properly with the correct fibers.

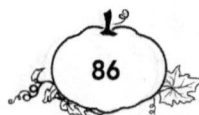

> Remember: the right balance of diverse bacteria must come first. Then you need to feed those bacteria the correct fibers.

Some people over-feed the same bacteria by eating and drinking the same things every day and instead of creating a gut landscape rich in diversity, it's like a farmer who only grows one crop. As the mono-cultured bacterium grow in number, they dominate and push out the others so there is less diversity.

All of the names and required amounts of all the gut bacteria are still being discovered and as this field of research grows, treatments are fine tuned. We already know the names of the bigger players and importantly we know:

- ☐ What they do
- ☐ How they benefit health in the correct numbers
- ☐ How they hinder health if the numbers are too high and
- ☐ What it means for our health if their numbers are too low or not present at all

Yes, your symptoms are the way you suffer, but to me your symptoms are telltale keys to solving a mystery.

> Whilst there are differences in symptoms for each patient, they show me the presence or absence of different types of bacterium. This is especially evident with my patients who experience excess tiredness.

Fatigue Patterns

My chronically tired patients who can describe their fatigue in intricate detail – they know their own pattern all too well, because they constantly endure it. When they tell me about a particular fatigue pattern and how it feels in their body, I listen very closely for the clues.

Fatigue presents as different patterns. These patterns can be described in many ways, for example:

- Consider a fatigue pattern with an energy drop at a certain point in the day, particularly after food or in the absence of food or if feeling stressed.
- In contrast to those who feel bone-tired all day or
- The aching fatigue of the immune compromised or the patient struggling with a virus.

These different patterns are each driven by a different bacterial presence or absence, requiring a correction to return the gut to its homeostatic balance, and thus the ability to generate energy. In this way we see fatigue as a symptom of a gut problem rather than something to be put up with. If you struggle with fatigue, finding the energy to get some help can see you caught in a vicious cycle. Little steps are a great way to get started.

Pain Patterns

The same principle of gut diversity can be applied to pain patterns.

- Pain can present all over the body in muscles, organs and joints and seem to stay in one place, like a throb or ache.
- Pain can be widespread and present all the time but moving.
- Pain can feel either dull or sharp, a constant presence or on and off in one spot, with a changing intensity throughout the day.

Headache and Migraine Patterns

Headaches and migraines are another specific pattern. The type of headache and when they come on, and the level of their intensity, always alerts me to a different bacterial imbalance.

Rash Patterns

Rashes signal to me that the cause is coming from the gut when the rash is always there but changes in its intensity, or it breaks out and then vanishes, only to reappear in another part of the body. These mysterious variations unnerve the patient but steer me towards a healing solution in their gut.

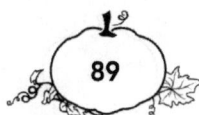

In addition to understanding the symptoms and presentation of how each person experiences 'their' specific rash-pattern, I also want to know what is happening with their poo.

The patterns give me clues about what is likely happening in the gut, and information about the poo gives me the keys to solve the pattern.

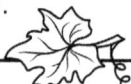

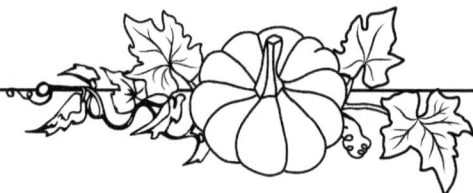

Hannah's Migraine Story

Hannah presented with extreme migraines making her a regular at the local hospital emergency department at least once a month. She'd be given various medications and ongoing prescriptions for pain management. This was all very front-line triage management, and the focus was to manage the pain on the day, so that life could return to almost normal. I say almost normal because the underlying cause was always still lurking. It was only a matter of time before another flare-up would occur.

I knew that to help Hannah, I had to help her out of this vicious cycle, so I began to shift things by asking her if she had ever heard the saying, *"If you always do what you have always done, you will always get what you have always got."* I informed her that the gut answer to any problematic health pattern is to change!

I am grateful when people choose to invest in the type of testing that I recommend. I often see people who are very sick and want to get on top of ongoing ill-health. They invest the money, the time, and the effort and they do really well. They feel so much better than they ever did before. But it's not unusual for a patient to ask, *"When can I go back to my normal diet?"*

It's hard to accept that what was 'normal' was the pathway to ill-health and the 'old normal' has to be replaced by a new normal.

After testing Hannah's poo, I discovered a complex bacterial imbalance that was producing toxic metabolites. These metabolites were cooking her body from the inside. Her liver wasn't coping with the over-production of toxins and then, on top of that, the regular pain-medications were putting further strain on Hannah's system and also suppressing vital bacteria.

It felt like we had to turn around the Titanic. Meaning the changes that were made now, would not be felt for a while, but they needed to be made and a new course needed to be set, and continued for quite some time.

One of the recommendations I made based on Hannah's stool report was,

"Eat more vegetables, more fibers, more variety. Eat more vegetable skins and peels, and more fibrous stalks that you normally throw away."

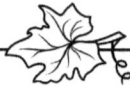

I sometimes feel like I am on repeat with this advice for many people. This is a habit to build slowly, park it in your mind now, and leave it there, so if ever in any doubt, eat more vegetables.

The other recommendation I often make based on a **stool** report is to stop all sugar, fruit, glucose and lactose.

These are the big guns when it comes to feeding the same bacteria over and over. Remember that unhealthy dietary patterns result in bacterial overgrowths where one or two species of bacteria dominate the entire colon, which is soon expressed as symptoms.

I use the nutritional panel on food as a guide and restrict all sugar content to under 6 for every 100ml or grams.

This level is low and will help you to stop feeding the same bacteria. It's time to learn a new healthy respect for sugar (even fruit). It doesn't mean never again, but it does mean never again dominating your gut bacteria. You may fear you will forever suffer sugar cravings, but you won't, as these are a symptom of gut imbalance and instead you will have greater energy.

It isn't what you do every now and then that causes a problem, it is what you do every day that creates the cornerstones for your health (or your ill-health).

It's time to be realistic and honest...

- ☐ Are you a processed sugar fiend? Or...
- ☐ Do you eat copious amounts of fruit (including dates) and think you're doing yourself a favor?
- ☐ Or do you drink lots of fruit juice to feed that sweet tooth?

"Fruit juice is healthy, isn't it?" I hear you ask.
"Fruit?" You exclaim even more loudly and hopefully.

Remember, it's what you do every day that is the foundation upon which your state of health is built. Fruit is still a sugar that feeds those specific sugar-hungry bacteria. And while I'm appearing to be a kill-joy, don't forget that alcoholic drinks contain lots of sugar! Again, I am not saying never again – but for a therapeutic period of time it may need to go – and when it comes back – it is a treat for occasions and celebrations.

Upon following my advice, I received this feedback from Hannah:

"I am feeling a lot better in the gut"

"Bloating is all gone"

"Increased energy"

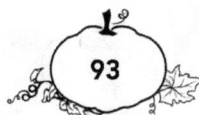

"Increased focus"

"The headaches are less frequent. When I do have one now, it doesn't last as long, and I recover quicker."

"Once I started following this protocol, there have been no more trips to the emergency department – yeah!!

I know we are on the right track, and it is not the time to stray from the path…"

A Word on Pain and Excess Weight

Typically, I see a recurring picture with pain and high-end pain management. This is also the case with excess weight gain. In these cases, there is always an imbalance of the key performers – the balance of Bacteroides being gram-negative and the Firmicutes being gram-positive.

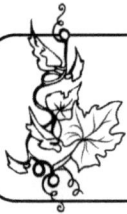

> Bacteroides should be the most abundant anaerobe present in the colon.

These are the fat burning gram-negative bacteria, which need to be present in a variety of species. A range of between six to seven species provides a great start. These are the bacteria responsible for producing the short chain fatty acids (SCFAs) from vegetable fibers.

SCFAs are a major source of fuel for the colonocytes. Bacteroides are important for fat emulsification by providing what is termed alpha-sitosterols – these are required to support this process.

The second most abundant anaerobic bacteria that need to be present are the Eubacteria. These provide the beta-sitosterols needed for fat emulsification and absorption.

Alpha-sitosterols are like the left and beta-sitosterols are like the right hand, both these guys are needed. Inside the human digestive system, the lack of one of these major players will alert me to fat malabsorption, which will play out as cholesterol issues and hormonal dysregulation among other things.

How far along you are in your bowel dysbiosis (the extent of bacterial imbalance present in the large intestine, or colon), especially when it comes to these two key players in fat malabsorption, will be further evidenced in the rest of your pathology results.

Pathology results often show low levels of the fat-soluble vitamins A, D, E and K, along with high cholesterol and hormonal changes. In particular, hormonal changes include low dehydroepiandrosterone (DHEA), which is the building block of all sex hormones. Other possible impacts also include changes to the rest of the sex hormones such as oestrogen, progesterone, and testosterone. It is further possible thyroid hormones (T3 and T4) or pancreatic hormones, such as insulin, may be adversely impacted if these two groups of bacteria are out of balance or not present.

Lisa's Pain and Weight-Gain Story

I consulted with Lisa in 2020. I saw very high levels of pain and weight-gain, which stemmed from a Bacteroides to Firmicutes imbalance. The metabolites being produced from her bacterial overgrowth were making high (unhealthy) levels of lipopolysaccharides (LPS), hydrogen sulfide, acetate and lactate. One of the key symptoms here is the production of smelly gas. This is a key sign you have bacteria producing something noxious so please don't succumb to feeling embarrassed or self-conscious, just take note of foul-smelling wind or stool. These are symptoms, rather than characteristics about yourself.

This bacterial imbalance all added up to very high acidity levels with loads of pain and weight gain that would not shift, no matter what Lisa ate. Despite several strategies that had been suggested by well-intentioned healthcare professionals, Lisa was stuck and I knew that nothing would change until her gut imbalance was addressed.

Once I shed light on the inflammatory factory that was occurring in Lisa's gut, together with her physician, we were able to prescribe a very short dose of a specific antibiotic that targeted the bowel. This was followed with natural antimicrobials to do the rest of the gut work. I recommended following this with an alkalizing regime and a dietary protocol that stopped feeding the bacteria with sugars including lactose, fructose, glucose and even carbohydrates (these break down to glucose).

The protocol for Lisa also started with a flush, which helped reduce the fecal load in the gut from the onset. Vegetables and bone broth also featured in her recovery diet.

The Outcome

Improved pain management and weight-loss followed for Lisa who said, "I feel as though I'm back in control of my weight and body again."

Tip: Love your Anaerobic Bacteria Hard!

Bacteroides should make up 90% of the bacteria present in your colon. It is the fibers in our food that feed the Bacteroides, which produce essential SCFAs. As mentioned, these are a major fuel source for your colonocytes. SCFAs help keep us warm, protect the fragile inner surface of the gut, to prevent us from becoming unwell from nasties such as *Salmonella*.

There is no probiotic available which contains Bacteroides as they cannot exist outside the gut. So, we have to eat the right foods to feed the varied subspecies of Bacteroides and keep their levels high.

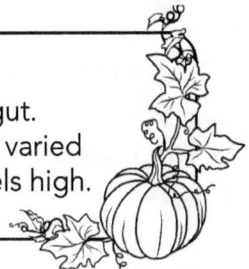

The Eubacterium species are the other main anaerobe. These should be second most abundant after the Bacteroides. Eubacterium play an important role in fat absorption and therefore hormone regulation.

Unfortunately, many probiotic supplements contain key bacteria that can also be in overgrowth and contribute to digestive symptoms. If you've been taking a probiotic for some time and are experiencing any symptoms, try coming off the probiotic for a while, especially if you've been relying on the probiotic to keep digestive symptoms at bay.

Needing a probiotic is also a sign something is out of balance in the gut. The questions that need answering are:

1. Are you taking the right thing to solve the imbalance? Or,
2. Are you suppressing or adding to the problem?

Perhaps it's time to test your poo and understand what your gut really needs to solve the imbalance and stop the symptoms *and* the cause!

To Test or Not to Test?

The Question of Parasites

Bacteria can be brought into balance, but parasites have no place in your gut! The tell-tale sign that parasites are involved is when symptoms are extreme and something has to be done – and fast!

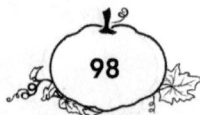

> There is no sweet spot for parasites. They simply should not be present at all – they've gotta go!

They are often detected via standard medical testing; however, many doctors are loath to recommend treatment as it's often ineffective.

My concern about parasites being allowed to persist, is that they leave a path of destruction in the gut that is very hard to treat years after the initial infection.

Having the special armoury to treat parasites quickly is one of my specialties.

> The two big nasties that are hardest to treat are called *Dientamoeba fragilis* and *Blastocystis hominis*. Just their names may send a shudder down the spine.

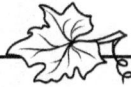

Parasites – *Dientamoeba fragilis* and *Blastocystis hominis* Symptoms

I often see persistent diarrhea in patients with these parasites. This sometimes regulates back to a firm stool and creates confusion by giving the appearance that you are all clear. In longer-term patients, it can develop into constipation.

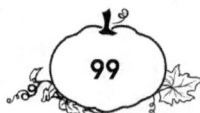

Parasites can also be responsible for:

- Eczema and other skin conditions.
- Fatigue and low iron.
- Headaches and migraines.
- Bloating and wind.
- Triggering autoimmunity.

Parasites at School Story

Some time ago, I began seeing a spate of parasites in young children who all lived in the local area.

Each child presented differently, but often with at least several of the following:

- ☐ Extreme eczema
- ☐ Weight loss
- ☐ Failure to thrive
- ☐ Erratic mood swings
- ☐ Fatigue
- ☐ Poor concentration
- ☐ Persistent diarrhea
- ☐ Malaise
- ☐ Aches and pains and even
- ☐ Anal leakage

I was busy making up herb mixes, requesting specific antibiotics in extreme cases and providing corrective support supplementation.

Every child improved with treatment and the parents reported that all symptoms disappeared.

I loved getting these messages and calls from parents who were relieved to see their children thriving again. However, within a short period of time, the children began to experience a return of symptoms.

It was perplexing. One day I had a regular catch up with another local naturopath, and dear friend, Anita Toi. It's always great to catch up with a colleague to swap notes, hear another perspective and support each other.

She was reporting similar cases, and when we dug deeper, cross-referencing our notes, we found that all the children involved were from the same school. Together, we decided to approach one family that was involved at the school committee level. We raised the question about whether the water supply of the school could be contaminated.

We described the recurrence of symptoms after successful treatment and highlighted the fact that all the children we had independently treated, attended the same school. Once the children were clear of symptoms and went back to school, the symptoms returned in every case.

It wasn't a simple process, but because of the persistence of the families involved, and our evidence, the matter was looked into by the school. The water was tested and proved to be contaminated. The local authorities stepped in to address the issue and with repeated corrective treatment, the children all recovered.

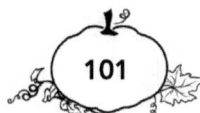

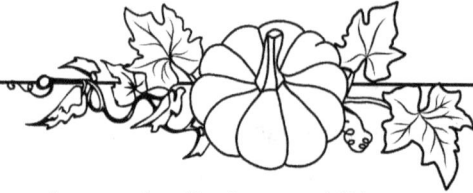

Why did the water supply affect some children and not others?

You may wonder why some of the children were infected and others at the school were not, especially as all children at the school had access to the same water.

It's a good question and needs to take into consideration:

1. The volume of water each child potentially drank.
2. The individual susceptibility of each child's immune system, and
3. The quality of each child's stomach acid.

All in all, it was a good outcome for the children, their families, the school and the local community.

Stomach Acid

Everything we eat and drink has to pass through the pit of hydrochloric acid (HCl) that's produced in our stomach. Healthy levels of this acid should be sufficient to kill off any potential intruder, such as a parasite trying to get into our system. This wondrous mechanism usually offers enough protection.

However, some people have insufficient stomach acid. This is called hypochlorhydria and among a number of other reasons, it may be more commonly due to:

- Low histamines
- Low B12
- Stress
- The presence of *Helicobacter pylori* and
- Some medications

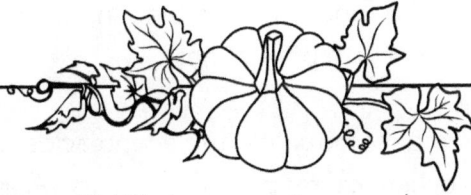

Boiling water will kill these nasties, so always boil water when travelling or camping, even for teeth brushing and especially for washing vegetables.

Allergies

Allergies fascinate me. Why do some people's immune systems overreact to environmental triggers, such as pollen, or animal hair, or dust, and other people's don't?

In my years of studying allergies and working with hundreds of patients with allergy symptoms, it's very satisfying to address the root cause of these triggers. At the time of writing this book, new evidence has recently come to light which relates to the gut and the production of amines in the gut being caused by certain bacteria.

Recent research suggests that the gut is a hidden source of amine production that has until now been overlooked. Previously, we concentrated on blood results and radioallergosorbent or RAST testing to alert us to the allergenic triggers. A RAST test uses a blood test to check for IgE antibodies to find out to what substance/s a person may be reactive. Reactions can vary from mild to life threatening. It now turns out that gut bacteria are often responsible for food sensitivity and intolerance due to the production of amines into polyamines.

This is due to the decarboxylation of amino acids. This is a fancy name for the biochemical reaction that occurs when amino acids are broken down inside our digestive system. These amino acids come from the proteins we eat.

Foods that are high in protein include:

- [ ] Eggs
- [ ] Meat (both red and white flesh)
- [ ] Fish
- [ ] Dairy products

These provide our digestive system with a pool of amino acids, which have many different roles and destinations inside the human body.

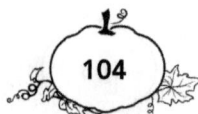

When our digestive systems work effectively, the amino acids break down and don't travel down to the large intestine, and it isn't a problem. However, when digestion is compromised these amino acids become the substrate for the bacteria to act upon.

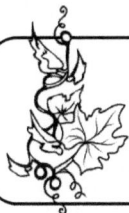

> This then becomes the hidden factory of amines in the gut, triggering allergy responses and sensitivity.

This can include changes in blood pressure which can explain mysterious dizzy spells or a racing heart.

It's not enough to just improve digestion by giving support to the production of stomach acid or pancreatic enzymes. This is helpful, but not the whole picture. What is also needed is to moderate the amount of protein in the diet, reduce overall histamine consumption (see appendix III for a list of these foods,) support digestion with enzymes and to alkalize the environment inside the body. Such strategies offer what I call a multi-pronged approach.

This turns down signs and symptoms of excessive reactivity at every level inside the body. It also takes the burden off the body's immune system.

For some patients it's not the protein that is the problem, it could be other various gut reactions that are specifically associated with lactose and glucose, or fructose and sucrose. These are all different sugars present in foods including fruits and some vegetables. A stool test result is important to provide clarity on the specific cause.

Alkalizing

One of the reasons I love alkalizing so much is that it limits this reactivity and therefore turns down sensitivity in the gut. Alkalizing limits the production of amines and polyamines, as well as reducing the impact of gut reactions due to other causes.

> The solution for allergies is all about which bacteria are present and knowing how you feed these bacteria with your food choices.

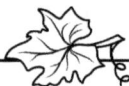

Change the substrate (the foods you eat), and you can change the acidity and improve other signs and symptoms along the way.

When a patient presents with a very strong allergy picture, I know it's likely there is a secret amine factory in the gut. Just like any other factory, it can't keep up production if it's starved of the raw materials, and the amine factory will close down, restoring your gut to balance.

My Daughter's Allergy Story

I have a healing story that features my beautiful daughter (yes, I'm biased) when she was only 10.

The start of the downturn is vivid in my mind. It was a hot summer night and, as we live at the beach, we cooled off by having a swim in the ocean. My daughter was still in the water when she began vomiting. That was January, school was about to start and there was so much happening. She was moving into a new grade; we had a new kitten and change was in the air.

School started and the symptoms became worse.

Most days, the school would ring, asking me to pick up my daughter from the sick bay. Sometimes I would say to my daughter, *"Don't go to school today, sweetheart,"* because I knew she wasn't going to last more than two hours.

Starting at a new school, new grade, and also missing so much school, meant that making new friends was harder for her and she began the year on the back foot.

I made an emergency appointment and the doctor suggested appendicitis; the symptoms were there. As I was more concerned about my daughter at the time, I didn't acknowledge that I had a few of the symptoms too, all except the major one, vomiting. It didn't dawn on me at first that there was a link.

Blood tests were done for my daughter, and I asked the doctor to include a few extra things I wanted to see that they normally wouldn't test.

Later that night I received one of those dreaded calls. You may know the type of call I mean...when the doctor calls after hours, you know they're about to tell you that something is not okay.

The doctor informed me that my daughter's inflammatory markers were elevated, and I needed to get her in to see a surgeon for an appendectomy as soon as possible. This was alarming, but also playing in the back of my mind was that I felt the same *AND* I definitely did not have appendicitis.

The next day, after another sleepless night, I made a time to see my own doctor who knew me well. I told her I felt the same. I raised the question about whether it was possible that my daughter did NOT have appendicitis. I have always been one to question everything. It drives my kids crazy at times, but it is my nature. So, the doctor asked me: *"What do you want to do?"* and I replied, *"I want to test my daughter's poo."*

I walked my talk and tested my daughter's poo (and mine at the same time).

It turned out that we both had two parasites! And our gut bacteria imbalance was almost identical (her results were slightly worse than mine).

By this point my darling girl had only been to school for about three weeks of the entire term. Fortunately, at this young age they catch up fast and the most important thing for her to do was heal.

It was coming up to Easter and we had to do the toughest gut protocol ever (we called it boot camp) it included no sugar, not even fruit. It was hard not giving Easter chocolates that year, but the stakes were high.

My daughter's blood work looked like she had chronic fatigue and as a sufferer of this invisible fatigue syndrome myself, I did not wish that on her, so we threw everything at recovery for both our sakes.

The thing about kids is they are like super balls; they bounce back. We killed those nasty parasites by addressing the rest of the microbiota balance with diet. We did some alkalizing and pumped up her energy, and she was healthy and got straight back into the swing of things without missing a step.

Adults on the other hand have more work to do and while mine and my daughter's reports looked almost identical, our road to recovery was quite different.

The one thing that children and young adults have on their side is growth hormone, which helps to mend and fix many issues fast. However, from the third decade on, the amount of growth hormone produced recedes and our capacity to repair is reduced. Consequently, adults just don't bounce back at the same rate. We have to work harder and for longer. It doesn't mean we don't get there, but extra effort is needed.

Once we have the poo test results, the next step is of course, the gut protocol. The gut protocol not only addresses the symptoms, but most importantly, solves the cause. Guess what Chapter 5 addresses? Yep, you guessed right, the gut protocol.

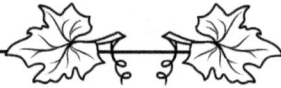

Chapter 4 - Take Home Highlights

FACT: Research is now showing that autoimmune conditions start in the gut!

- Consider your symptoms – what are possible triggers for your symptoms?

- A word of caution – it's best to avoid strict diets which exclude key food groups.

- Your gut is more than just a poo making factory – it is in fact home to many different types of bacteria which work hard to feed and fuel your cells and your body!

- Your mood, sleep, energy, aches, pains, skin, hormones, body weight, ability to heal and much more – all depend on the balance or imbalance of bacteria inside your gut.

- There is no sweet spot for parasites as these do not belong in your gut – seek treatment from a professional!

- Feed your Bacteroides and SCFA production – consume a wide variety of vegetables every day.

- Alkalizing is a key way of restoring balance to your digestive function.

- Symptoms, such as bloating and allergies, always have a pattern – seek professional help to unpack what your pattern means.

- You're never too old to heal your gut, however the younger you are the quicker you will bounce back due to higher levels of growth hormone.

THE GUT PROTOCOL

7 STEPS TO A HEALTHY GUT
& VIBRANT LIFE

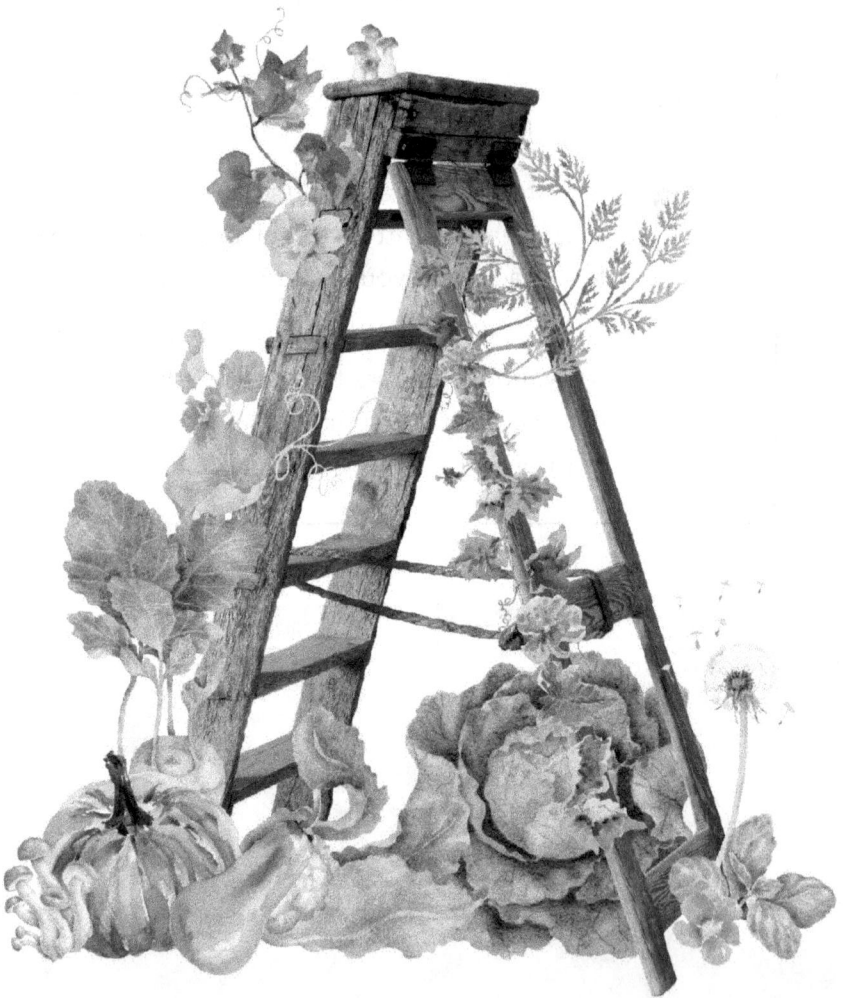

The process revealed

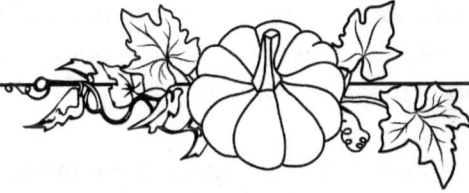

Heather's Heavy Metal Speech Loss Story

Back in 2013, I met a patient called Heather, who had a major life crisis. One result was that Heather lost her speech. I couldn't imagine what she and her family had been going through as they were awaiting results to confirm if she had suffered a stroke. Heather's husband, John, was understandably anxious, in a brief telephone conversation I simply asked him, *"Do you have a plan?"*

John replied, *"No, not really."*

I smiled gently, *"Well, I do."*

When a patient walks into an emergency department presenting with sudden loss of speech and a tooth abscess, the first thought is to investigate for stroke. To an integrative medicine practitioner, such as myself, along with investigating stroke, the next question is about possible leakage from mercury-amalgams which could have led to toxicity within the brain.

We worked together as a team to unravel the mystery of what was happening in Heather's body to produce such an extreme symptom, such as loss of voice.

My approach has always been to work with the evidence provided and, in this case, there was so much going on, we tested everything… and I mean everything!

Once I had the information, I interpreted the results and outlined a course of action and the steps that needed to be put into place. At one stage we all reached a point of overload. It was too much information to deal with and we needed all heads on the challenge to make use of the information.

The first step was the chelation of heavy metals in her system, and most importantly her brain. Chelation Therapy is a way of removing heavy metals from the blood, particularly mercury which is a poison. I didn't have everything on hand to support her in the detoxification process, so I took her to a treatment center where I knew she would be fully supported.

During the car trips back and forth to the center, I learnt how to communicate with Heather by asking the right questions and then listening to her cues. Heather would type on an iPad if she needed to provide detailed information.

At this early stage, managing the results of a stool test was too much for Heather and the team around her to focus on. I knew that her gut would take the brunt of the detox so we focused on the chelation of the heavy metals first. Once the detox was done, we would then correct Heather's gut imbalance.

Sometime into the heavy metal treatment regime I dropped by her house with some supplements. Heather came outside to meet me and spoke two words: *"Thank you."*

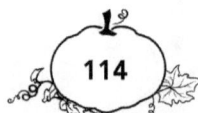

I never imagined that two simple words could be so beautiful and so meaningful. I dropped to my knees in tears, overwhelmed with emotion. This time, I was the one who was speechless!

Fast forward to 2019, and we were ready to re-test Heather's stool to manage the final steps of her healing journey. It was time to flush out high levels of bacteria that were in overgrowth and implement a gut protocol to reset her system to achieve balance.

> It was like taking a nice deep breath to focus back in on the important stuff; commencing the process of restoring, optimizing and then maintaining Heather's gut microbiota.

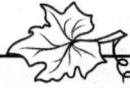

After all the turmoil and intensity of the past, the timing was perfect for Heather to focus on the protocol I prescribed. She was delighted to lose weight, gain energy, and have sustained focus. She adopted a healthy mindset towards the foods that were nourishing her body.

Best of all, her speech fully returned I cannot tell you how moving it was to hear such an articulate woman free to fully express herself. Heather's journey didn't end there, as she fed herself her true nutritional needs, she began to find a deeper truth within her and gave voice to this truth in her words and actions in her life. Truly amazing Heather!

My 7 Step Gut Protocol

From one person to the next, the gut protocol can be very involved. The protocol will *always* involve changing the diet, as it is important to stop feeding the bacteria that are in overgrowth.

Step 1: Stop Feeding the Imbalance

This simply involves not eating those foods causing the problem in your gut! Almost universally this includes those high in added sugar. It may also include eliminating fruit, foods containing lactose and removing alcohol. It will be ok, you can do it, I promise.

If you have been hosting and overfeeding a bacterial or other type of microbial overgrowth and you want to change how you feel, what you do and what you eat need to change too. This also includes all the alternative sweeteners high in sugars, such as dates, maple syrup, rice malt syrup and honey. Please also check individual labels on foods such as: tinned vegetables, pickles, tomato sauce and other foods, which may be high in either natural or added sugars.

Step 2: Change the Gut Environment

If you have a predominance of gram-positive bacteria there will be a lot of acid being produced. You can immediately gain the upper hand by alkalizing. I use alkalizing smoothies (refer to the recipes in the bonus recipe chapter at the end of this book) and alkalizing mineral powder.

Step 3: Suppress the Overgrowth

This is what I call the kill factor, which sounds rather harsh, and of course, all our gut bacteria is good – we just need everything in the sweet spot of homeostatic balance.

We kill off the excessive bacteria to make room for other bacteria to colonize. Diversity is essential in the gut. I will often use a natural antimicrobial. I have a few I like to use depending on the bacteria in question. I use these in a pulse therapy done one week on and one week off. During the 'killing week' I will go hard, and this often produces die off – so don't be discouraged if you initially feel much worse before you feel better. It's not the most pleasant sign of progress but when die off occurs, I secretly rub my hands together with glee. We are on target and getting results!

I follow this with a week of restoring the gut to a better balance, which may mean taking very specific probiotics, if indicated by the stool sample analysis. When overgrowth is extreme, I'm guided by the expert advice from my consulting microbiologist (I love your work Henry!) and use antibiotics that are specific to the bacteria in overgrowth. I'll suggest this for short sharp targeted suppression, and then follow up with natural antimicrobials.

This step always involves implementing specific dietary measures. I then return back to the 'kill factor' the following week. I'm not in favor of using either antibiotics or herbal anti-microbials long-term. Both are powerful and have their place. However, if you are taking these types of products long-term you will suppress many diverse species, which is the opposite of what you need in your gut.

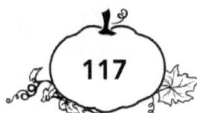

When I speak to people who take antimicrobial or antibacterial herbs long-term to look after their immunity or to assist gut function, I often see suppression of important bacteria. This is the case with people taking herbs such as olive leaf extract or oregano oil for example. There are many powerful herbs, and in my armory, they are big guns to be used sparingly.

If you're looking to improve your immune status, I do recommend nutrients and, naturally, I prefer to test. The balance or imbalance of bacteria in your gut is unique to you, so it's important to get a stool test and have a unique protocol prescribed just for you.

Step 4: Support with the Correct Nutrients

While the gut microbiota is a miraculous factory making myriad nutrients from different metabolites, such as coenzymeQ10, folate and many amino acids, my work involves rebalancing the gut. It's like I am re-educating the gut how to function properly. As the saying goes "feed a person fish and you have given them a meal but teach a person to fish and they can feed themselves for a lifetime." This step adopts the same concept. While improving the body's own ability to produce nutrients, I am also supplementing nutrients at the right dose. This is done only for the period of time necessary to support the body until it can step in and do this naturally – reset and forget!

Step 5: Replace Bacteria

Step 5 may involve using only very specific probiotics, if any at all. I admit, I'm not the biggest fan of purchased probiotics, which is somewhat unusual in the naturopathic industry. I share the same goal as my naturopath colleagues, but I aim to create the solution within the gut.

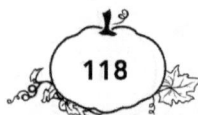

Even *Lactobacillus spp.* and *Bifidobacterium spp.*, which are gram-positive can contribute to metabolic acidosis, inadvertently compounding the problem. Remember, your gut is unique and your solution is unique and the poo test allows us to be more targeted and thus more effective in healing your gut.

When I analyze stool test results, the pattern of overgrowth is a recurring situation for almost every patient typically corrected without the need for probiotics. On those rare occasions when I recommend probiotics, I am looking for D-lactate free probiotics, which will not contribute to the biogenic amine load, and will also not further contribute to the acidic load in the colon.

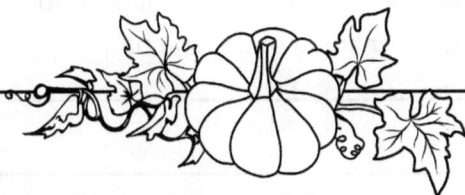

A Side Note on Fatigue and Chronic Fatigue

This last point is very important to remember, especially in the case of fatigue, particularly chronic fatigue. The conversion from the D-lactate to the L-lactate form occurs in the mitochondria inside each cell. Remember in Chapter One 'Mary's Sugar Addiction Story'? It was here I first introduced you to ATP. ATP is made from the food we eat and provides energy to power every cell in our body. This includes providing energy to our muscle cells so we can move, our nerve cells so our brain can function and much more. ATP is also made inside our mitochondria.

A Side Note on Fatigue and Chronic Fatigue

You may also recall that a build-up of D-lactate is very problematic. This is because excessive D-lactate slows mitochondrial function, which reduces ATP or energy production. The result of this is fatigue. In addition to impaired energy, metabolic acidosis will also contribute to urinary acidosis, adversely affecting kidney function, protein digestion, and not to mention undermining the health of the inner lining of the colon.

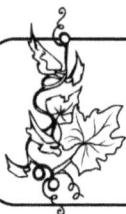

The stakes here are high, so I am very fussy when choosing probiotics for my patients!

It's no wonder I bang on about alkalizing. (Refer back to Step 2 of the gut protocol.)

Step 6: Feed your Gut the Right Bacteria Fodder

The right bacteria fodder means fiber, fiber and more fiber to feed your bacteria. This in turn feeds your colonocytes, which is a fancy name for the cells that line your colon.

Soluble and Insoluble Fiber

Essentially there are two main types of fiber:

1. Soluble and

2. Insoluble

As a general rule, most people need to eat more insoluble fibers, but not in cases where the gut is too deficient in the bacteria needed to breakdown these insoluble fibers.

> Where insoluble fiber is not well tolerated, bloating is the key gut symptom.

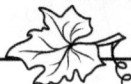

In this situation, the focus must initially be on consuming soluble fibers only as a preparatory step in a two-step process. Soluble fibers (see list below) are water soluble and come from plant pectins and gums. They become sticky and gel-like when mixed with water and can help slow down the digestion of food. The gut initially needs to be filled with these fibers before it can handle any insoluble fiber. Only then should you slowly begin to re-introduce insoluble fibers.

Soluble fiber-rich foods include:

(See Appendices for a further list)

- Avocado flesh
- Peeled pumpkin
- Peeled carrots
- Peeled zucchini
- Peeled sweet potato
- Peeled turnip
- Peeled cucumber
- Very well de-strung celery
- Peas
- Brussel sprouts
- Okra
- Peeled beetroot
- Psyllium husks
- Black beans
- Lima beans
- Navy beans
- Pinto beans
- Kidney beans
- Sunflower seeds
- Flaxseeds

Insoluble fiber comes from:

☐ The plant cell walls, including cellulose, hemicellulose and lignin. These are found in the skins and peels of vegetables and fruit as well as the bran portion of the wholegrains. This is important for the bulk of your stool but more importantly these feed up the bacteria that you need most in the gut.

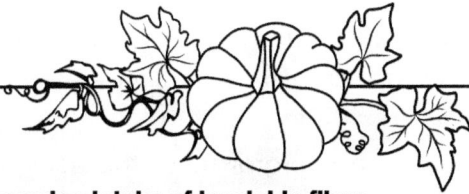

Tips for increasing intake of insoluble fiber:

🎃 Eat more insoluble fibers from vegetables including skins, peels and fibrous stalks.

🎃 Look to increase the variety of vegetables eaten.

🎃 Look for more seasonal varieties.

🎃 Include whole grains, nuts and seeds with skins and husks.

Bone Broth

In most cases, I also recommend drinking bone broth and also meat broth for healing the gut lining and building good bacteria. However, I do not *always* recommend bone broth. I have had some patients who do not benefit from this. Bone broth is not necessarily a panacea, as it does not substitute the benefits that you get by eating more vegetables.

I do not recommend the consumption of fermented products including fermented vegetables, sauerkraut and kimchi. Added to this list is kombucha, kefir, yoghurt and even sourdough breads or fermented protein powders.

The reason for this is along the same lines as the probiotics and even herbal antimicrobials. These foods are medicinal and when used in a dose-specific way are well placed *for the right person* with a particular gut microbiota picture, but ad-hoc use as a general health practice can cause imbalance.

Most patients have an overgrowth of the acid-producing and amine-producing bacteria from these food substances, which then further contribute to gut symptoms, allergies, neurocognitive symptoms and fatigue.

For those people who do a stool sample and present with allergies, fatigue and neurocognitive symptoms, I often see species such as *Corynebacterium spp.* and *Leuconostoc spp.*, and *Weissella spp.*, as well as *Lactococcus lactis*. These species are found in very high amounts in many fermented products.

Diversity is key

I have mentioned this before. But in my experience, many people are trying to find the single ONE thing, or 'easy' solution. They grab on to the latest fads or the superfood culture citing: "This or that is good for me, it's *THE* answer."

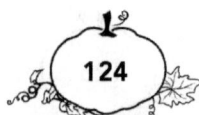

People then tend to just do that one thing. We've become addicted to health regimes.

Forgive me if I repeat myself here, I do it out of my wish for you to be the healthiest version of yourself…

> Everything has a threshold, and gut homeostasis has a sweet spot.

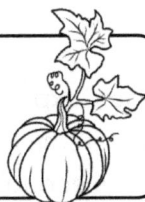

There is even a limit to how much broccoli you should eat daily… *I'm just sayin', variety IS the spice of life.*

Next, a word on dietary change and why it can be so hard

Food Cravings: 'Me' or 'Not Me'?
There are times when we crave specific foods, sugar in particular is the key culprit here. Quite often for some people, there is an element of feeling like the urge for sugar is beyond their control. If you hear yourself say, *"I should know better,"* you are correct but beating yourself up won't help.

Make no mistake about it – it's not always in your head. There is an element of…

"It's not me, it's my bacteria."

Your Gut Bacteria Influence Cravings

It's been proven that bacteria will reward you for feeding them, and potentially influence and even exclude the desire for foods that would support their competition (microbe competitor, that is).

When explaining this phenomenon, I describe the battle and what it's going to take to gain the upper hand. Even knowing this fact is enough for some people to resist the temptation of an ice cream at the end of a hot day, or that chocolate biscuit with a cup of tea or coffee. We are trading immediate gratification for a deeper lasting reward in the form of great health.

Step 7: Support Digestion with Enzymes and Bile

Our last step is an important step to enable your digestion to be properly supported from the stomach and pancreas. It ensures your foods, and especially proteins and fats, are being broken down into smaller particles for absorption.

To this end, I often support patients by using stomach acid supplements containing hydrochloric acid (HCl), pancreatic enzymes and especially trypsin, pepsin and bile.

The Importance of Bile

Bile is a vital fluid containing electrolytes, bicarbonate-rich, cholesterol, phospholipids and bilirubin.

It's a critical part of digestion and absorption of fats and fat-soluble vitamins in the small intestine. I can often pinpoint a lack of bile flow and also fat malabsorption via pathology results, your stool results and signs and symptoms.

> Common signs of poor bile flow are shown in a floating stool and/or an unformed stool.

Many waste products, including bilirubin, are eliminated from the body by secretion into bile and elimination in stool. Secretion into bile is a major route for eliminating cholesterol. It's interesting that you need to consume fat to stimulate bile. I recommend consuming good fats like olive oil daily. I also recommend lemon juice in water to help stimulate bile flow.

Bile acids have a detergent action on particles of dietary fat which causes fat globules to break down. Bile acids are fat carriers and are also critical for transport and absorption of the fat-soluble vitamins.

Bile is also important for the breakdown and removal of other toxins including biotoxins and used hormones.

HCl (Hydrochloric Acid)

In the stomach, HCl's primary function is to maintain a sterile environment and begin to breakdown proteins. HCl contributes to disease resistance by destroying most ingested pathogens and bacteria that are on, or inside, the foods you eat.

It's one of the reasons some people suffer negative effects from ingesting parasites and others don't. (Remember the case of our school children and their polluted water supply where not all students became symptomatic?)

> It is all a matter of the robustness of the acid pit in your stomach.

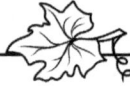

Acid Reflux, or GERD/GORD?

Low stomach acid production is far more often a problem than high acid production. This is despite a recent estimate by Australian researchers that Aussie doctors prescribe drugs to supress stomach acid production in 95 out of 100 patients suffering from acid reflux, or GERD.

Recent estimates put the prevalence of GERD in Western countries, including Australia, as impacting between 10-20% of the population.

In my clinical experience, many of my patients taking drugs to supress stomach acid production come to see me because they continue to experience digestive symptoms lower down in their digestive systems, even though they are taking anti-reflux medication according to the instructions.

My approach is to detect and treat the gut cause to effectively resolve digestive symptoms.

Part of this approach is to let my patients know I will be treating them for low or less than normal stomach acid production. Hypochlorhydria is the technical term for less than the normal amount of acid, while achlorhydria is the term used to describe what happens when no stomach acid is being produced at all both conditions are extremely concerning.

Time and again, many of my patients also present with an intolerance to certain foods. An important reason for this is that they lack enough stomach acid to chemically digest the food they consume. A lack of HCl in the stomach will cause an incomplete conversion of the proteins from food into amino acids, which causes real problems in the colon, as already discussed above.

More often I see an over-abundance of gram-positive bacteria in these patients. This type of overgrowth contributes to the over-production of acid throughout the entire gut and most importantly the colon, rather than an over-production of acid in the stomach itself.

The next chapter starts with my no bullshit heath tips to potentially address these challenges and the many other symptoms we've discussed so far.

Chapter 5 - Take Home Highlights

FACT: Healthy stomach acid production does more than help to break down the food we eat – it also contributes to disease resistance by destroying most ingested pathogens and bacteria that are on or inside the foods we eat!

- If you have either a complex medical condition or complex symptoms, it is best to work with a practitioner, or a team of medical practitioners to get yourself well.

- Stop over-feeding the same bacteria – especially avoid foods high in natural or added sugars, including sweetened tinned food, pickles, sauces, fruit, all sweeteners (except stevia), as well as lactose and alcohol.

- Change the gut environment – remember to alkalize.

- Supress the overgrowth – remember to avoid trigger foods.

- Support digestive function with the right herbs and supplements – work with a practitioner to get this right.

- Replace the right bacteria but be specific – work with a practitioner to get this right.

- Feed yourself the right fibers – improve your soluble and insoluble fiber intake.

- Support your digestion – consider your stomach acid, pancreatic enzymes and bile production.

- Refer to the recipes in the bonus recipe chapter at the end of this book.

- Anti-microbial herbal medicines and nutrients for immune support may have a place, but are best used under the guidance of a practitioner.

- Use probiotics either not at all, or under the guidance of your practitioner.

- Consuming good fats like olive oil daily and lemon juice in water to help stimulate bile flow.

Chapter Six

KARLENE'S GUT HEALTH TIPS

LITTLE THINGS ADDED TOGETHER MAKE BIG CHANGES

This is a checklist of things to do and tick off

Start improving your gut health today by replacing foods and habits that are currently hindering you rather than helping you to feel great.

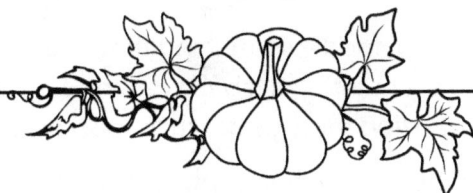

Karlene's Top 10 Gut Health Tips

Whilst my treatments are person-specific, there are some universal health practices that you can start on right now:

1. Buzz a green smoothie every day to alkalize and provide nourishing vegetable fibers. Change what you put in the smoothie regularly (refer to my top recipes at the end of this book).

2. Above all else, eat way more plant-based foods – enjoy a mostly plant-based diet.

3. Eat something different once a week, if ox tongue takes your fancy, then go for it! Or maybe it is sardines on a salad, or oysters, organic liver pate or perhaps try okra for the first time…test your adventurous spirit.

4. Consume fat for bile flow. I like high-quality olive oil with lemon, the perfect combo for your bile to flow. Or maybe it is fresh avocado that excites you today.

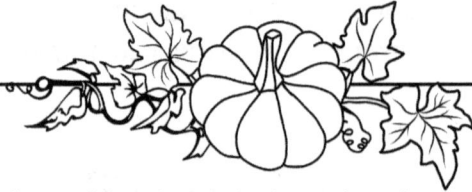

5. Go for real food – something that doesn't have to provide a nutritional label. I call this **Low Human Intervention** food, rather than food products.

6. Clean out the kitchen cupboards and change what you put in your shopping trolley from one week to the next. Variety is key. Don't worry, the family will just think you have gone gourmet.

7. When reading a nutritional label make sure the total sugars are under 6 per 100 millilitres or per 100 grams.

8. Add bone broth to wet or liquid food. When purchasing meat, think 'BONES!' Buy beef bones, lamb bones, fish bones, or chicken frames and slow cook them with lots of vegetables, then eat the vegetables and the liquid when cooked. Make sure they are organic, wild caught, or grass fed. Add a dash of apple cider vinegar to enhance de-mineralisation of the bones.

9. Vary the foods you eat. Rotate a food so it is eaten once every four days. This helps prevent allergies developing as you are not consuming the same proteins and fibers every day.

10. Do a **Flow check-up**. As results filter through I can help with what still needs tweaking (refer to the next chapter.)

Allergies

I was recently in deep discussion with my naturopath friend and colleague Kristi Grbin. We both commented on the different phases of our lives, and what we now know that would have served us better. One of the main discussions was about how we had both inadvertently created allergy problems by over-consuming one or another supposed 'health foods.'

My ninth gut health tip, the four-day rotation of food varieties, stems from this reflection on my own experience as well as seeing what thresholds have played out for my patients over the years.

My Love Affair with Oats

I loved oats. They nourished my mind, body and soul. I thought I was doing the right thing when I consumed them almost exclusively during stressful exam periods. All because I knew they would sit well, keep me calm and feed my brain. Sadly, I over did it and now I have a strong IgE reaction to oats. While it is not quite at the level of anaphylaxis, it is still a big reaction none the less.

> My take home message here is that everything is dose-dependent. Everything (and every food choice) has a sweet spot.

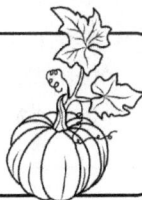

Imagine a farmer who grows only one crop, year in, year out, depleting the land through monoculture, compared to a permaculture approach where all the plants are complementary and create a healthy ecosystem without depleting the soil. That's your gut – increasing variety is the way to go.

Daniel's Dryness Story

Daniel presented with fatigue, pain, anxiety and depression. So, we completed a stool sample. Daniel was experiencing a standout digestive symptom of dryness throughout his entire system. The difficulty with his treatment was that it involved suppressing the Clostridia species of bacterium.

These bacteria are a bit like a macadamia nut; they are tough to crack! That's a mom joke! With the correct anti-microbials, coupled with the right probiotics, a reduction in numbers can occur. There was lots of to-ing and fro-ing with Daniel as we refined his diet and tried to introduce and increase his intake of fresh vegetables.

We needed to ensure he included lots of variety. We worked through many different cooking styles but the results were intermittent, he had good and bad days and he needed to make daily variations to his diet.

After testing, and interpreting the results, I often see my role with my patients as a teacher. I show them how to read and interpret the signs and then give them the tools to adapt and adjust based on those signs.

Daniel had come a long way and certainly there were health benefits. In particular, sleep was a key sign for Daniel that reflected the composition of his gut microbiota and also changes in acidity.

> At one point it felt like he had hit a plateau and no matter what we did, progress had halted.

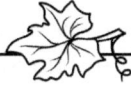

It was at this point that he elected to re-focus by doing another stool test.

This was a brilliant decision. While the results showed there was still more work to be done in other areas, the key area we were addressing had completely resolved. This included the Clostridia being reduced to a healthy number, whilst the Bacteroides had markedly increased. The battle had largely been won.

I was so pleased Daniel had the re-test. Re-testing helped to determine the cause of the remaining symptoms and the treatment could be adjusted accordingly. Even though work needed to continue in other areas, he was well and truly on the right path.

Lou's Ulcerative Colitis Story

Ulcerative colitis (UC) and Crohn's Disease are two Inflammatory bowel diseases where symptoms can wreak havoc with the flow of life. The symptoms are so extreme that the patient often plans their whole life around a "what if" scenario. These people need to know where the nearest toilet is always…I even had one client who installed a toilet in his van just to be covered. Planning is often everything in the lives of those with inflammatory bowel disease.

Lou was a patient who worked in the health industry as a Functional Nutritionist. Her knowledge of her condition and how to look after herself were extensive and she was doing a fabulous job. Her most alarming symptom was the regular occurrence of blood in her stool – which kept her in a cycle of worry, anxiety depression and fatigue.

Lou was on the front foot when she consulted me. She already had many of the answers, so the stool test was foremost. We needed this detailed report to spearhead the rest of her healing plan. As you may have guessed, the stool test results that came back from the laboratory were specific to Lou; the results reflected Lou's microbiota, but a troubling issue arose. Lou's specialist did not support the idea that Lou had an active role to play in her own healing process. The specialist advised Lou to 'accept,' or 'put up with' her symptoms because *"this is just your life"*.

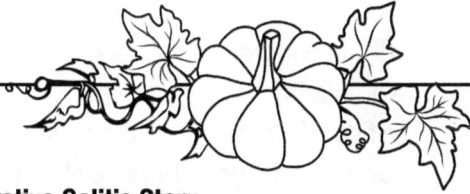

Lou's Ulcerative Colitis Story

Fortunately, Lou adopted a positive attitude and decided to be proactive about her health. She was resourceful and found a way to get the extra support she needed from her medical team and completed her protocol in full.

Lou's results at the 6-week mark saw:

- Bloating and inflammation all gone.
- Decreased pain.
- Reduced bleeding.
- Occasional loose stool (big improvement.)

Management is the key for both UC and Crohn's disease but certainly lots can be done when you truly know your specific results and work steadily towards balance.

Building Bacteroides Species

One of the things I address frequently based on stool test results is the imperative to build up Bacteroides species. These are the all-important SCFA-producing bacteria that are needed most abundantly in the distal colon, or the far end of the lower colon. These bacteria feed colonocytes and break down fats, essential for our good health.

Sadly, many of my patients' stool test results show an insufficiency in both variety of these bacteria and also in total numbers. Bacteroides need an alkaline environment to proliferate and grow. We often significantly reduce or even wipe them out by consuming a highly acidic diet, or in times of high stress or even from over-exercising.

In order to renew these bacteria, I emphasize the importance of alkalizing and then provide a list of a variety of vegetable fibers and wholegrains, as well as bone broth to build them back up again. However, it is always multi-factorial, and stress reduction is also a key part of creating a healthy setting for these bacteria to thrive. I'll talk more about stress in the next chapter.

Bacteroides can only grow and exist in the gut environment – so I can't give them to you in a supplement. It is all done in situ – in your gut – like a science lab. So how do you know when you are growing them successfully? The answer is in how you feel… meaning no bloating, ease of digestive function and awesome poo.

Where to Next?

At a certain point in a patient's protocol journey, when they reach a stage where the evidence shows that they are well on their way to better gut health, I ask them to pause. I also ask them to consider how far they've come and…where to next?

The overall function of the gut has improved by this stage, and they may no longer notice all the big or little symptoms that niggled at them when they first started. There may be some work

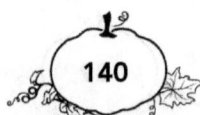

still to do, but the health momentum is building. That's when it's time for the Flow Check-up, which I'll address in the following chapter.

The Flow Check-up helps to determine tweaks and adjustments as symptoms ease and results are achieved. It lets us know what has rebalanced and what still potentially needs more work.

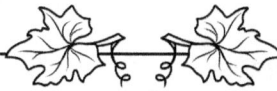

Chapter 6 Take Home Highlights

FACT: it is possible for your body to develop an IgE immune reaction to one or more foods through repeated exposures over time – it is wise to avoid over-consuming specific foods.

- Use my 'Top 10 Gut Health Tips' to start improving your health today.
- Swap out problem foods and habits for healthy alternatives.
- Be mindful – you can create allergies if you over do one particular food!
- Be resourceful when implementing the right support for you.
- Change up your diet regularly and use a variety of different cooking styles.

- Bacteroides are your best friends – you cannot have too many.

- Feed your Bacteroides – consume insoluble vegetable fibers every day (refer to lists of foods to focus on inside this chapter.)

- Remember to pause – consider just how far you have come and where to next?

- Consider symptoms that remain – determine tweaks and adjustments needed (see next chapter.)

Chapter Seven

THE FLOW CHECK UP

HOW TO KEEP THE GOOD RESULTS COMING

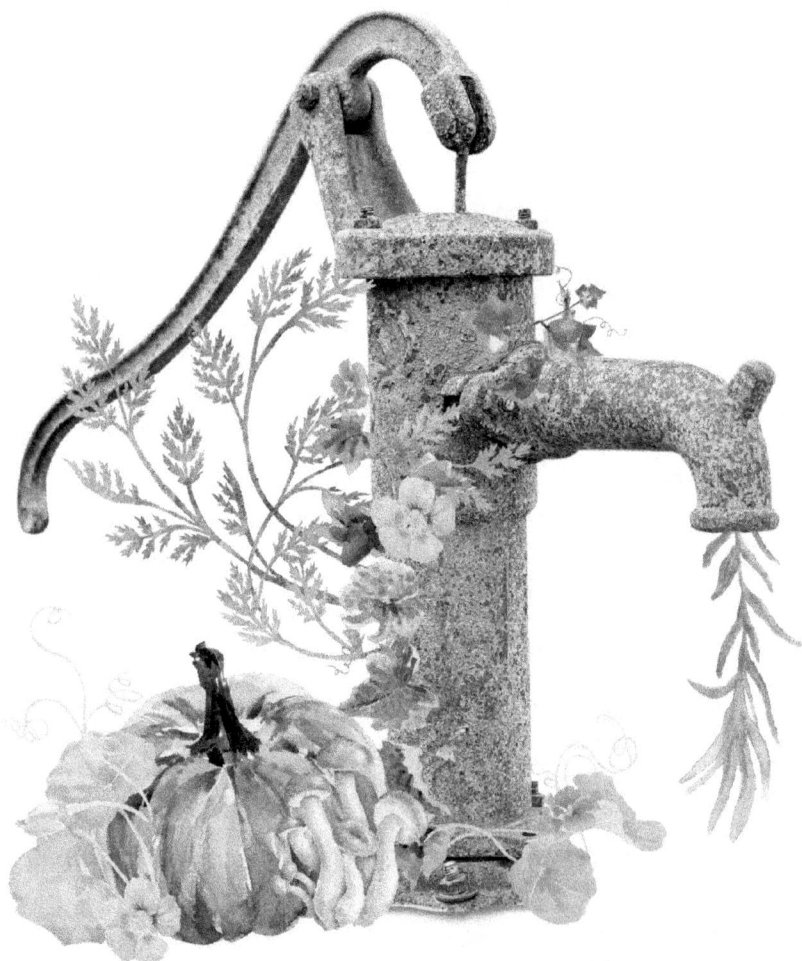

Review and staying true to your path
– watch for self sabotage

The Flow Check-up is an important step on the path to optimal gut health.

If you have already taken steps to have a stool test, and you are undertaking a gut protocol tailored for your unique needs, you've probably already achieved some great results.

The next step is to identify what has or has not changed. There will be some things that will need to be pursued further, while other aspects of the protocol will need to be adjusted to meet the changing symptoms and gut balance.

One of the easiest ways to do the Flow Check-up (see chart below) is to check your original list of symptoms. There is also the option to re-test. The Flow Check-up involves:

1. Start by tuning into your gut for symptoms - these are the messages you're constantly receiving.

2. Checking your poo every morning by comparing it to the stool chart.

3. Testing as things begin to change.

4. Noticing if something still doesn't 'feel' right when you tune in or look at what you deposited in the toilet bowl.

It's important to regularly check back in on your symptoms, and list and tick off what has changed. Sometimes it's good to keep a diary or even a spreadsheet to compare your progress. Even going so far as giving yourself a score on a scale of 1 to 10. Where these symptoms were sitting when you started.

As you progress you may see a pattern emerging. Perhaps the score gradually changes over the first few weeks, and you hadn't realized that you were feeling better. A bit like the frog in the pot that didn't notice the temperature rising – the daily improvements can be subtle but when you collect the data, it allows you the opportunity to reflect objectively on the improvements.

Sample: daily symptom collection chart including your poo report – (please see appendices for a detailed chart)

Sign/Symptom	What to expect	Your rating (1 to 10)
Wind, bloating, burping, reflux and of course your poo	The average person farts about 4-15 times per day, (the average is 8). Maybe that's spread throughout the day, or maybe you do that over 10 minutes. Windy symptoms are a sign that something is fermenting, and it is time to address what is causing this.	
Pain levels	Different for everyone	
Poo	Refer to the stool chart (remember the optimal poo is number 4 on the chart)	

Sign/Symptom	What to expect	Your rating (1 to 10)
Energy levels	Different for everyone	
Other		

There is always a golden nugget in every stool test report. That is, there is something that you need to learn and follow for the rest of your life as a way to keep your health on track. Sometimes we aren't looking for the nugget and so we miss this lesson, repeating it over and over again until we finally get it.

There are always cheat days and a way to undo any major indiscretion is to alkalize. I'll explain more in the next chapter.

Knowing what you can get away with and understanding what the signs are when you are heading in the wrong direction is crucial.

Remember the main thing to keep a close eye on is your poo, your number twos should be number fours.

Get curious about what your poo looks like daily and reach for the solution to everything…that solution is poo number four on my stool chart.

At this stage in your gut protocol, you may be thinking:

I hope this is over so I can get back to my normal diet.

Just a reminder, your normal diet was the problem! A permanent change in diet is a must if you wish to fix your health problems and improve your gut function. However, your diet needs to continue to change and evolve as your gut microbiota returns to balance.

Everybody is different so it is best not to compare yourself to others or to think *"Joe gets away with it – why can't I?"* In actual fact, you don't know Joe's story. Things may not in reality be quite as they appear. There is no point in drawing comparisons. It's best to get on with your own health journey and learn what you need to know to look after the exquisite body you have been gifted. Your body is telling you things you need to know by using little messages in the symptoms and sensations you experience from day to day.

Changes in symptoms will occur within weeks; however, it takes an average of three years on a new eating plan for the changes to be fully reflected in your microbiota. So, hang in there, you're worth it and those three years will pass by regardless, so you will be pleased you stayed on track!

Food as Medicine

Food is one of the most powerful medicines in the universe.

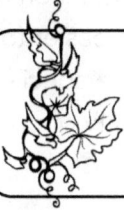

> What we eat becomes us – it is reflected in our skin, our brain, our heart, in our emotional and mental wellbeing and in every cell in our body.

Food controls our metabolism, memory, and sleep, as well as our psychology, our energy, our libido, our capacity to retain information and our intelligence. Food affects our mood, our compassion and tolerance. The impacts of our food choices on our health are way beyond just our energy and body weight.

According to Shawn Stevenson, food actually has the capacity to transform our society for the following reasons:

- Hypertension, diabetes and obesity are the top three killers in today's world. The human race needs help more than ever as our metabolic health is self-inflicted due to poor food choices. All of the top three causes of death can be influenced positively or negatively with a change in diet.

- Inflammation is at the root of most chronic disease states, and it is the decline of gut microbiota diversity that is contributing to major chronic health conditions in my view.

A rainforest analogy works well here. We need the large and the small growth for sustainability and not only are we looking at the possibility of endangered species we are also looking at extinction. Extinction is a very hard place to recover from. It is much easier to supress an overgrowth than it is to establish a species from nothing. This is the same for the diversity of our microbiota.

The decline of the gut microbiota has been linked to obesity.

The lack of diversity has been linked to increased health risk and susceptibility. Now more than ever the oneness with all things is paramount for us to maintain homeostasis with life itself; this is what nature intended and we are not separate to nature. Can you take a moment and consider how your forebears were deeply connected to nature and that as much as they would have loved electricity and a flushing toilet, their guts were healthier When we are out of balance with nature, this is when the symptoms begin. Can you begin to make nature a part of your daily essential greens?

Now more than ever we need to take better care of ourselves and our gut otherwise we are not fit enough to respond to other threats to our health and wellbeing.

I realize that this perspective is not necessarily among the popularly held beliefs in healthcare today. However, I am reminded of the Nobel Prize winners, Warren and Marshall, for the discovery of *Helicobacter pylori* and the treatment for gastric ulcers.

They first encountered resistance to their theory, until Marshall published results of self-induced infection after deliberately swallowing the bacteria to produce symptoms. Then they followed up their discovery with successful treatment. Sometimes, this is what it takes to provide an alternate hypothesis to health.

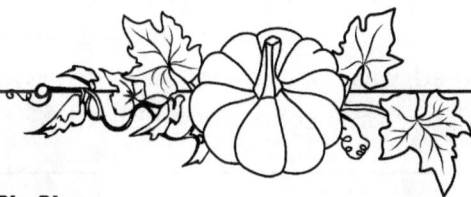

Penny the Pig Story

My son's kindergarten had quite a menagerie, including a pet pig.

Anyone with a pig as a pet will know how pigs are incredible. However, this rescue pig was stressed, and she had developed a type of psoriasis. As I looked at this beautiful creature, I remarked how in humans we look to the liver when we see psoriasis, so I was intrigued to find out what was happening with her diet.

It is quite hard to keep up with the sheer volume of food that is required for a full-size pig to thrive. The scraps from the kindergarten simply weren't enough. So, our darling pig had other sources of food coming from a variety of scraps and handouts from the community. Basically, she was being fed every scrap of any food from whomever supplied it. There was no consistency in quality, only lots of quantity.

When I spoke with her owner, I mentioned that we needed to find a higher quality, high volume food source for Penny the Pig. So, the owner spoke to a local organic vegetarian café and secured the scraps daily from the tables and the kitchen. Anything that was not consumed, was put aside for this much-loved pig. Within three months Penny's skin condition vanished!

> The quality of food really does show from the inside out!

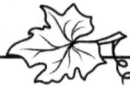

Self-Sabotage

These days many people are highly educated and aware about what to eat, but why is it that we just don't do it? Is it self-sabotage?

Matt's Acne Story

Matt was a young patient with acne. He did so well on his specific protocol and his skin ended up looking flawless. Everyone was so happy, and his mother told me that they tore up the Roaccutane script that the dermatologist had written. This was great news for his gut because this well-known prescription medication for acne has a way of drying all your mucosal surfaces, leading to further problems in years to come. Often these longer-term problems occur in the gut, but also the bladder and lungs too. In fact, all your internal mucus membranes can be impacted.

The tricky scenario when helping young adults is their social life and the need to fit in and feel accepted. Peer pressure and fear of missing out (FOMO) means it can take courage to go against the flow of the social group, to say no to the pizza, or decline chocolate, alcohol, and other tempting goodies.

Matt struggled with missing out on what the other guys could eat without it affecting their skin (It was affecting their health in other ways of course). This attachment to food in social settings led him to feel pressured into conforming to the group. He felt the resentment of *'Why me?'* As a result, Matt decided the pressure made it too hard to maintain the protocol.

At this young stage of his life, he was not willing to continue with the changes to his diet for the long term, which would sustain the improvements in his skin. He chose to return to taking the medication. Both pathways achieved radiant skin, however, one path required immediate sacrifices to achieve the outcome. Time will tell if there will be long-term consequences from taking the medication. Sometimes it's a matter of timing and at least Matt knows that he can always return to the protocol when he is ready.

Naturally, health is always your decision. Are you prepared to do what it takes to get the results you want? Sometimes our self-confidence has taken a hit because of our health struggles. Let me reassure you that you can change your diet and regain health and wellbeing, because your gut has its own solution. Change is always possible, and make sure you focus on taking things one day at a time and celebrate your milestones along the way, confirming your progress!

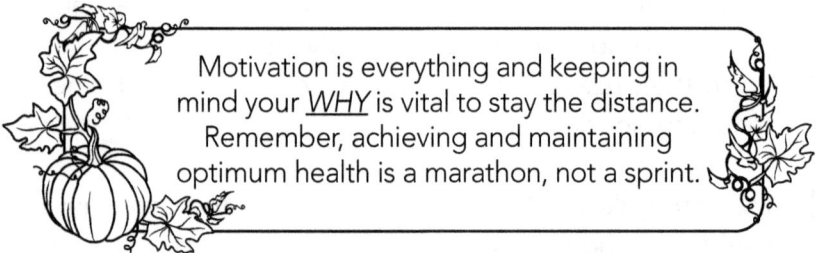

> Motivation is everything and keeping in mind your _WHY_ is vital to stay the distance. Remember, achieving and maintaining optimum health is a marathon, not a sprint.

A Moment to Consider STRESS

I call stress, the great un-doer.
Unmanaged stress and long periods of stress without a recovery

plan, play a major part in your gut microbiota balance. It's like the chicken or the egg scenario as we need a balance of key bacteria to help combat stress including:

- *E. coli*
- *Lactobacillus* and
- *Bifidobacterium*

These bacteria are the main players in healthy GABA production. GABA, or gamma-aminobutyric acid, is an important brain neurotransmitter that helps with maintaining calmness. GABA's main role in the body is to reduce the activity of neurons in the brain and central nervous system. It helps with relaxation, reduces stress, promotes a more balanced mood, alleviates pain, and aids sleep. Other effects of GABA also include lowering blood pressure.

So, GABA helps combat stress. When stress is not well-managed using appropriate recovery periods, the effects of stress on the body causes a drop in pH making the body more acidic. This in turn can kill off the all-important Bacteroides species, cause an increase in *sugar hungry bacteria*, and also a drop in the population of *E. coli*. Here is the catch-22 – *E. coli* is needed for the production of GABA.

The more you stress, the more this nasty downward spiral occurs:

1. There's reduced *E. coli* in your gut.
2. The less *E. coli* you have, the less GABA you produce.
3. The less GABA you produce, the more stressed you are.

Do you see where I'm going with this? It's a vicious cycle, so make sure that in addition to changing your diet, that you change how you manage stress. Seek out professional help or download meditation and mindfulness apps that will offer guided stress reduction programs. And listen to your gut – what is your gut trying to tell you about your relationships, your job, and your life. Sometimes we need to detox from a lot of toxic influences, at other times we need to get better tools to manage stress.

Chapter 7 - Take Home Highlights

FACT: it takes an average of three years following a new eating plan for the changes to be fully reflected in your microbiota – hang in there, you're worth it!

- Use the Flow Check-up – review your original list of symptoms.

- What has improved – see how far you have come.

- As your symptoms and gut balance change – adjust your protocol.

- Continue to check your poo against the stool chart every morning – before you flush.

- Work with a practitioner and retest as things change.

- Know your golden take home nugget – what is it *you* need to learn and follow for the rest of your life?

- Be aware of your own self sabotage patterns – get help from a practitioner if needed.

- Stress is the great un-doer of good gut bacteria diversity – put strategies in place to manage your stress!

Chapter Eight

YOUR NEW MAP TO A HEALTHY GUT & VIBRANT LIFE

KNOWING YOUR TRUTH IS KEY

This chapter contains some magic and a very personal message from me.

Your gut protocol isn't a punishment, it is a correction.

Our goal is to live a rich and vibrant life and health and wellbeing is the winning strategy!

The gut protocol doesn't have to dominate your life, the steps simply need to be in the back of your mind, like a trusted friend, letting you know you are on the right path and doing okay.

It is inevitable that life will throw curve balls your way. It happens to all of us. The curve balls are sometimes expected, like the Christmas season, or a birthday that triggers you to stray from your path. Other curve balls can come in the form of unexpected bad news or the death of a loved one, this is life.

Day-to-day stresses may be the thing that catches up with you by the end of the week.

Whatever life throws at you, know your shit!

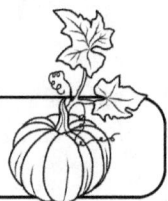

Having a reset meal will help get you back on track. When life gets a little out of hand, having a reset meal to pull it all back into alignment you move quickly back into the flow.

A Personal Message from Karlene To YOU:

Please take a few moments to reflect and allow me to speak to the entirety of you directly, including the cells of your body, the most stubborn symptoms and your inner voice that calls you to heal.

To all of this, I say:

"My darling, I am so sorry that you have had to suffer.

I know it can seem like it is unfair that you try so hard and yet you suffer. I know sometimes you wonder, what is the point?

Have you learnt anything from your suffering? Has this suffering told you what it likes? What it prefers? Can you hear what it wants instead?

Are you listening to your body's symptoms, the messages it tries to share with you? Do you feel the internal calling, to discover what you need to do to begin healing? Are you ready to discover the ways in which you need to care for yourself?

Are you aware yet of what your body needs you to eat to repair itself? Do you know the answers, but struggle? Do you try, and then falter?

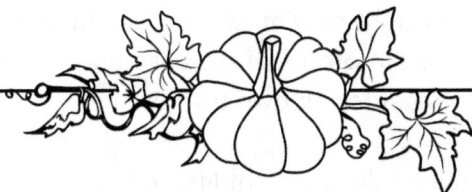

Do you hear your body's call to move? Do you know the signs that your gut, your digestive system, sends you? Are you listening yet? Are you ready to hear?

Dear one, your body is trying to communicate to you about your gut balance. Your gut health is reflected in your symptoms and your wellness. Your gut health is even reflected in your mind, and the quality of your thoughts.

Hear me when I tell you that your gut health reflects your energy levels and your passion for life too.

What has your body tried to tell you? What are you willing to do for your body? Are you willing to forgive your body? Your body forgives you. Are you willing to love your body back to health?

Take a further few moments to reflect and ponder your gut truths. Make some notes and then reflect upon your answers and insights.

It's much bigger than your gut right? It's your healthy and vibrant life! That's your birthright!

I trust that you now recognize that your Gut Truth can set you free – Free to just, 'Be'. Yes, that's our goal – just be You! By being true to yourself, you are in alignment, whereas if we betray our own truth, either in thought or diet, we are out of alignment and we will soon have the symptoms of dis-ease and anxiety to show us that we need to reset to our own true path.

Please claim your healthy, vibrant life and without trying, you will inspire others to do so and reclaim their truth. In this way, as you bring your best self to life, the world can only benefit – yep we're changing the world one gut at a time!

That's Good Shit!

YOUR RESET MEAL

You are not a robot and so it's neither a crime nor cause for panic if you fall into old ways. We simply anticipate that should this occur, we need to stop and correct, with what I call your 'reset meal'. Whatever meal you choose as your reset mechanism, refer back to that meal whenever you need a reset. Knowing your reset meal is like a beautiful mandala. Imagine you are the dot in the middle. What you learn throughout your unique protocol is what makes up the innermost circle of the mandala, the first ripple outward.

For some people their reset meal is:

- Bone broth soup with vegetables
- A small lean steak with a colorful salad
- Fresh fish (I recommend smaller wild caught fish) and a vibrant array of vegetables
- Maybe you do well with a vegetable-based dish served with quinoa or dahl
- Brown rice and a vegetable curry

- A crunchy salad with the protein of your choice
- Or perhaps it's one of my super smoothies that resets your mind and body (for a variety of smoothie ideas, refer to the bonus recipe chapter)

Or maybe for you it is not a meal, but rather:

- A staple supplement
- Digestive enzymes
- Or perhaps an alkalizing powder

> Your reset meal is gold, because you can always come back to it and use it to reset your mind and get cracking.

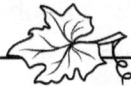

As the circles of the mandala ripple out you may remain stable, you observe your poo, give it a score and set your course to move forward with renewed confidence.

Your Personal GPS

Those of you of a certain age will remember carrying a book of maps in your car. In Melbourne, Australia we called it the Melways. In London, England they had the physical A-Z, and in New York there was the Hagstram guide for taxis and limousine drivers. When I grew up, it was with the Melways. Whoever sat in the front passenger seat of the car held the position of power! They held the map.

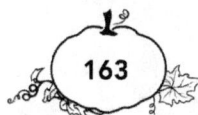

Now we all have Google Maps on our phones, which are GPS-driven. A GPS requires three points of reference for you to know where you are at any point in time. You now have your own digestive GPS, with your own three points of reference. It is all about how you read the signs and the choices you make given where each point directs your attention.

Your body's GPS and three points of reference include:

1. Your specific symptoms

2. Your poo as scored on the stool chart

3. Your energy

Be aware of the changes in the messages your body is giving you from day to day. The signs can be subtle so you may need to listen closely. For those who haven't listened in a while, the signs can hit you like a sledgehammer. Small one-off symptoms can appear like little red flags, or they may be like huge stop signs or the big one if you're not listening that says, "Wrong way turn back."

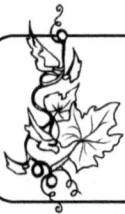

> The trick is to not only notice these little signs as they appear, but to then take action once you have noticed.

Chronic disease involves a significant microbiota change on the path to recovery. Resetting your trajectory to restore the flow is very important, so keep checking in with your main symptom list.

POST PROTOCOL BLISS

Throughout this process you will have accrued a lot of valuable information about you and your shit. This will serve you well when you put it into action.

Once you've got it worked out, when you know what to eat, how much you can eat, and know what your threshold is to reset, you often experience a feeling I call *'Post Protocol Bliss.'*

> This feels like you're Teflon coated, an inner confidence grows that feels loud and proud,

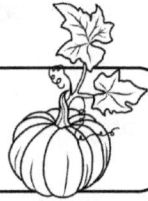

"I've got this…" it says.

But what if there is a little indiscretion here or a little slip up there? After committing to a gut protocol so stringently, life does need to get back to some sort of balance again, yes? Of course, it does. However, hopefully now many of the steps and choices you've made while doing the protocol, have become your new normal. It is, however, ok if you slip up or step out of line every now and then, but not every day or you'll be back to where you once were.

After doing your tailored gut protocol, your gut is now more resilient. You build resilience and you can handle a slip up more easily.

> The golden rule however is to simply remember to alkalize and then hit the reset meal.

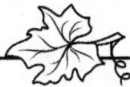

Problems arise when, after a slip up day, you don't alkalize, and you continue with more of the old ways and don't refer back to your reset meal. The quicker you reset, the more easily you'll avoid sliding down the slippery slope and getting to the stage where symptoms return.

Remember not to panic, no matter what stage you reset, you can save the situation from escalating. By this point you will have a feeling inside, a deep inner knowing that you have come so far, and you have learnt a lot. The benefits of feeling so great, the increased energy levels and being symptom free, far outweigh eating the treat food that triggered the symptoms every day, yes?

Hit your reset meal and you're back on track.

You now know what you need to eat to restore balance, so simply do that. Do it again and again until you step right back into that post protocol bliss. You do not have to go back to the beginning, you already hold the golden keys, just use them, and use them today.

GUT INSTINCT

Your gut is useful for more than intuition alone. Tuning into your gut and listening to its signs and symptoms, will always serve you well both in intuitive decision-making and mental, physical, emotional and spiritual health.

We need to navigate our path forward using our senses, checking in to reflect on symptoms, the signs and indicators every day. When this happens, we can make the little decisions about the smaller steps along the way rather than waiting for the big health crash.

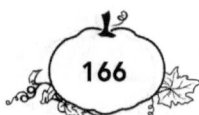

It's far kinder on your stress levels to:

- Tune in daily to your gut.
- Check your poo on the scale.
- Listen to the signs and symptoms your gut is sending you (the burps, farts, hiccups, reflux and the whole shebang.)
- Then use preventative steps and make reset decisions daily, rather than waiting till there is a debilitating health challenge to fix.

If you tune into your gut now, does it make sense to you? I suggest tuning into your gut daily to ask these questions:

1. Does this take me toward or away from my desired health goal?
2. Is it time to hit my reset meal to get on track?

A WORD ON SELF-SABOTAGE

Be aware of self-sabotage patterns and the influences and projections from those around you too. Just like my earlier story of our beautiful teenager Matt who made the decision to go off track due to peer pressure (that was Matt's sabotage mechanism), are you allowing anything to be your sabotage pattern too?

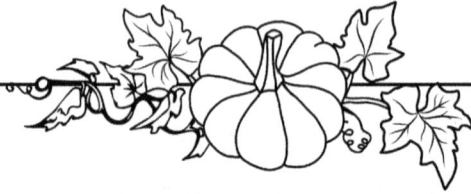

START IN THE KITCHEN – IT IS AN IMPORANT HEALTH INVESTMENT

The more you are prepared to invest in your kitchen preparation, the easier the path to recovery. It starts with:

- The time you allocate to planning, so you can make those key decisions about your health choices.

- What you stock in your cupboards.

- How you prepare meals.

- The ingredients you choose to put in those meals.

It does take time and effort to get your gut health in balance, but the payback is a long healthy life with lots of energy.

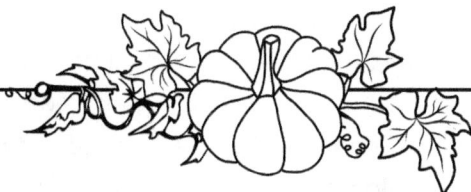

David's Autoimmune Story

David is a friend of mine who had an autoimmune condition affecting his liver. He followed the path I recommended and achieved a great result. My first recommendation for David was bone broth and high quantities of vegetables every day. I also suggested organic chicken to build up *Eubacterium*. There were many other steps in his journey, but after an initial stool test, this was where I suggested he should start.

Managing your health and what you eat is an everyday focus for people with autoimmunity. This was definitely the case for David who had been battling with this disorder for many years and, as he says, *"It feels like all my life."*

David's initial stool test results showed a dire situation. He had extremely high levels of hydrogen sulfide producing bacteria. These bacteria were cooking his liver from the inside out. A key sign of the production of hydrogen sulfide is a distinctive smell as mentioned in Chapter 4 in Lisa's story. As we progressed with his gut protocol, there were improvements along the way, but it was his third stool test results that provided us with the scientific evidence too.

Remember: it is NOT normal to consistently produce a strong or offensive smelling stool – take action today and seek assistance from your medical team and gut health practitioner as soon as possible.

In these results I saw a vast improvement in the balance. The levels of this bacteria had reduced significantly. However, his liver enzymes were still bouncing all over the place, and when he tuned into his "gut feeling" he was still getting the sensation that all was not as well as it should have been.

David was now consuming a plant-based diet, he was definitely providing all the insoluble fibers that the gut loves, but he was a self-confessed *foodie*. He always chose exotic fermented foods. As I mentioned earlier, these foods powerfully influence bacteria in the gut. For David, these foods included different sauerkrauts, kimchi, kombucha and sourdough. This wasn't helping as these bacteria were now in overgrowth.

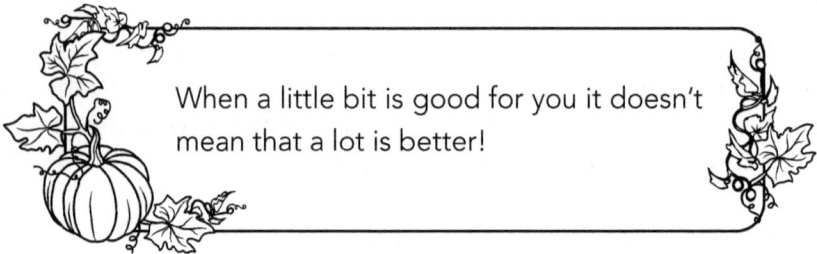

> When a little bit is good for you it doesn't mean that a lot is better!

He needed to drop the fermented foods fast.

Test results for David showed it was time to create some space in the gut. His gut needed a reset. I was quite specific with the best food choices for his body. These included: more leafy greens, colored vegetables, cruciferous vegetables and occasionally chicken bone broth and chicken meat. These were some of the things that would serve him well for the rest of his life. Now these kinds of changes are a big call for someone in their 40s, however, when you deal with a complex and life-threatening autoimmune condition, motivation can run high. So, in these cases, I become quite directive.

In a nutshell the changes included:

- Cruciferous vegetables such as broccoli, cauliflower, cabbage and brussels sprouts.
- Leafy greens.
- Highly colored vegetables such as carrot, pumpkin, beetroot, squash
- More seeds and nuts.
- Less grain – including less gluten free grains.
- Bone broth, and in this case specifically chicken.

I often suggest a 'set and forget' attitude with a certain repeating aspect that comes back in a stool report, especially if I see it in three separate test results. That really is a golden nugget that says very clearly, "*Just do this!*"

The more focus you are prepared to invest in your diet to provide the right substrate for your bacteria, the more benefits you experience in your quality of life and physical, emotional and mental health. You tend to notice:

- An ease in your gut function.
- No gurgles, no wind or bloating.
- Higher levels of energy.
- Being pain free.

🎃 Having good concentration, and

🎃 Restorative sleep.

All that is left to do is flush your number 4 poo away, then smile and get on with your day.

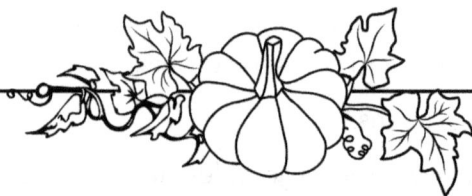

Here's a summary of important initial action steps.

Remember to:

a. Decide on a reset meal (and action it if relapse/ sabotage interferes.)

b. Check your number twos and look for the perfect number 4 very day.

c. Do a stool test if needed, definitely engage a professional who can interpret the results accurately.

d. Tune into your gut every day for signs and symptoms as well as listening to your inner knowing and instinct.

No turning back

As you have come this far with me on this journey, I'd like you consider that now you know stuff. You know to check in with your poo, tune into your gut, hit the reset meal and test, test and test.

When you choose to honor your 'Gut Truth' and strive for poo number 4, you take the first step towards a long and healthy relationship with your gut, your body, food and your health.

To make that a little easier, I've provided a bonus chapter with a few of my favorite recipes. You can also download many other recipes in a FREE recipe booklet as my gift to you at the link below.

In the Appendix of this book, I have added a range of resources. These include:

- A chart for you to track your digestive, mood and body symptoms.
- A guide to histamine foods.
- A guide to FODMAP foods.
- A start-up list of soluble versus insoluble fibers.

As I have referred to these foods and food components throughout the book, I thought it would be handy for you to have these crucial resources.

Remember to invest a little time in planning your food choices, clean out those kitchen cupboards.

Now you are free to get on with living your best life.
I know you can do it!
Go For It!
Love from
Karlene x

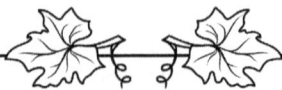

Chapter 8 - Take Home Highlights

FACT: you don't have to do it all alone – seek professional help if needed.

- Life will inevitably throw curve balls your way – accept this and move on fast.

- Know your shit – identify your reset meal and take action to reset and rebalance.

- Stock up on the right ingredients and plan your meals in advance.

- Alkalize daily to turn your health back around.

- Support your gut function with the right nutrients or supplements for your body's needs.

- Follow your gut Instincts to keep you uplifted and energized.

- Remember: use your body's GPS and three points of reference: identify your specific symptoms, rate your poo according to the stool chart and rate your energy.

- Use your personalized roadmap to stay on track and navigate your way forward!

FREE RECIPE BOOKLET

Access my favorite gut health recipes in the bonus chapter of this book. You can also download the complete recipe booklet with many more suggestions by accessing this link www.book.karlene.com.au/recipes

My Gut Health Recipes

FROM KARLENE GEORGIADIS

WELLBEING

The recipes I live by...
Easy to make, healthy, and fun

HEALTHY EATING

Snacks, Smoothies, and Dips
Breakfast, Lunch, and Dinners
Soups, Cakes and Slices
Special Occasion Food

EASY PEASY

I believe in keeping things simple, I've
tinkered with a few all time favorite
recipes and made them gut friendly,
yummy and fun.

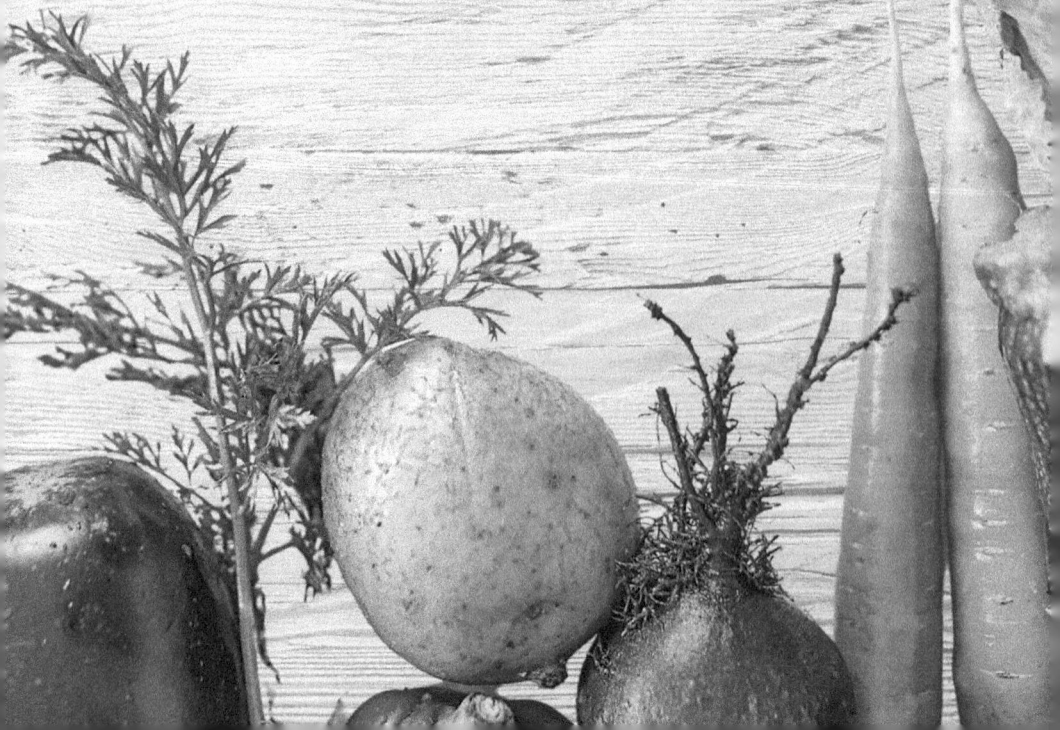

BONUS CHAPTER
RECIPES FOR GUT HEALTH
- STOP EATING CRAP

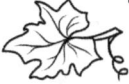

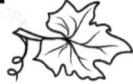

Included in this bonus chapter are some of my favorite and highly recommended smoothies, breakfasts, snacks, protocol salads, lunches and dinners (and special treats and sweets for the sweet tooth).

By request of my many patients, I have made this into a free mini recipe booklet that is available to download at:
www.book.karlene.com.au/recipes

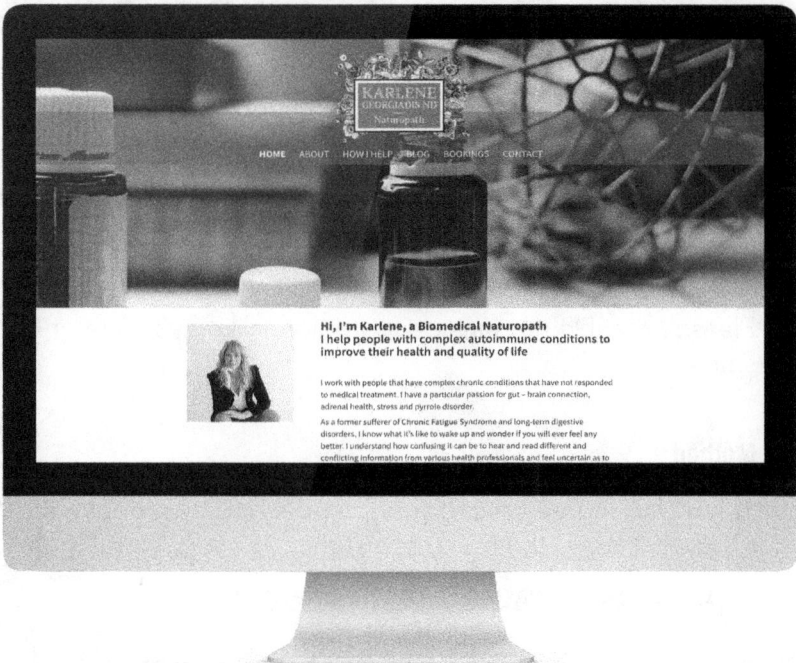

MY FAVORITE PROTOCOL SMOOTHIES

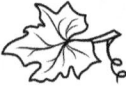

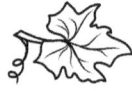

Alkalizing Smoothie – Buzz This

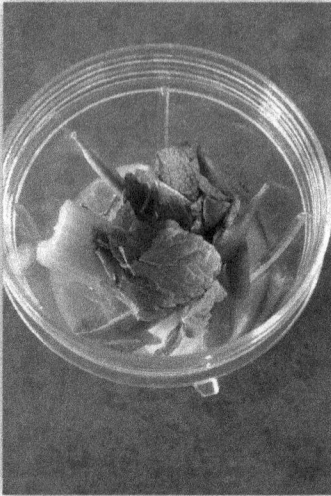

Ingredients

- 2 small celery sticks
- 2 baby cucumbers
- Some rocket
- Squeeze of lemon or lime
- 2 sugar snap peas
- Pea sprouts
- Or anything else green – change it up and add watercress, fennel, snow peas, beans
- Coconut water or filtered water

Please note: Do not include ingredients like fruit, kale or spinach.

Method

1. Add all ingredients to your blender and buzz until everything is the right consistency.
2. Consume slowly (as if you are chewing food.)

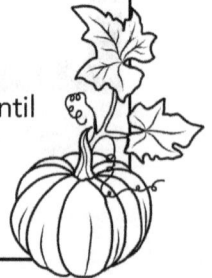

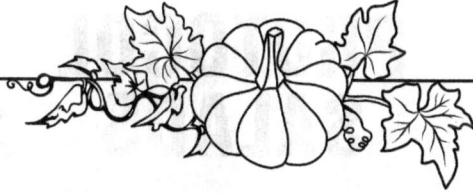

Protein Powder Almond or Coconut Milk Smoothie

Note: remember to check the almond milk and protein power labels for sugar content, which should be below 6 grams per 100 grams or 6mls per 100mls"

Add to your blender:

- Almond or coconut milk (check for sugar levels or make your own)
- Chia seeds
- Flaxseed meal
- Sugar-free protein powder containing either hydrolysed collagen proteins, hemp or pea protein
- Feel free to add stevia as sweetener if required

Method

1. Add all ingredients to your blender and buzz.

2. Consume slowly (as if you are chewing food)

Chia Pudding Alternative

1. Adapt the same smoothie recipe to make chia puddings.

2. Simply add more chia seeds then place the mixed ingredients in a jar. The ratio is 1 cup liquid :1/3 cup chia seeds.

3. Let it set overnight in the fridge.

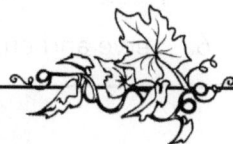

MY FAVORITE PROTOCOL SALADS

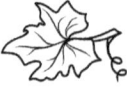 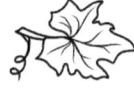

Tabouli Salad

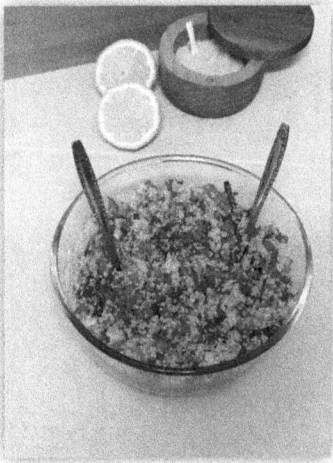

Serves 4

Ingredients

- 1 cup quinoa cooked
- 1 bunch parsley chopped
- ½ teaspoon Himalayan crystal salt
- 1 bunch chopped fresh mint
- Juice of 2 lemons
- 3 tomatoes finely chopped
- 1 small cucumber chopped
- 3 tablespoons of olive oil

Method

1. Place quinoa in saucepan and cover with cold water.

2. Leave to soak for 30 minutes.

3. Lightly simmer until quinoa is cooked (I wait for the little tails to pop out and the quinoa looks fluffy)

4. Drain and press out excess water.

5. Place all ingredients in a bowl and mix.

6. Serve and enjoy.

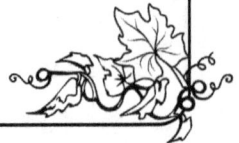

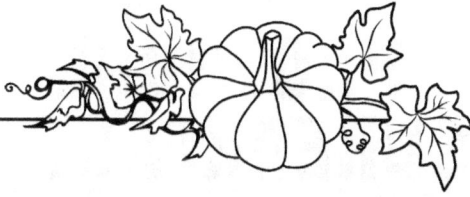

Reset Rainbow Salad

Serves 4-6 people

This is a favorite salad of mine that I make and eat as a quick gut health reset meal.

To me it is a rainbow in a bowl and so good for you. Of course, you need to be able to tolerate raw beetroot so if you are strictly FODMAP this would not suit your special needs.

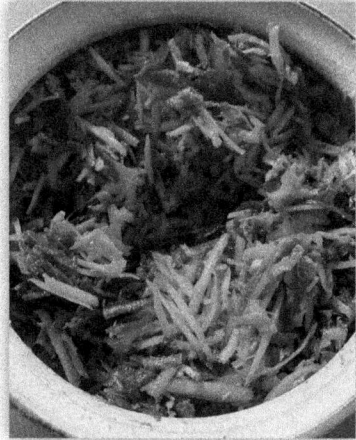

Ingredients

- 1 large raw beetroot (skin on) washed and grated
- 2 large raw carrots (skin on) washed and grated
- Large bunch of mint or coriander
- 1 heaped tablespoon of unhulled tahini
- 1 teaspoon of curry powder (I prefer madras)
- Pinch of salt
- Olive oil
- Apple cider vinegar
- 2 teaspoons black sesame seeds

Method

1. Add grated ingredients with chopped herbs and mix well.

2. Adjust salt to taste

3. Sprinkle with back sesame seeds and serve alone or with your favourite protein.

MY FAVORITE PROTOCOL SBREAKFASTS

Breakfast

- Eggs (your way). Add vegetables – you can go for roquette, mushrooms, and capsicum as the standard breakfast favourite, or, as there are no rules, get adventurous and use any vegetables that take your fancy
- What about a stir fry for breakfast?
- Or meatballs and vegetables?
- Zucchini slice
- Make my vegetable frittata and you have breakfasts for an entire week.

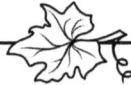

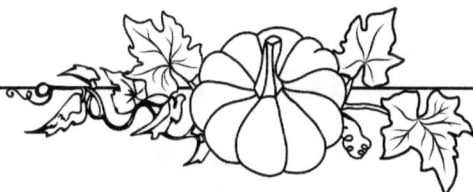

Porridge made with Quinoa Flakes

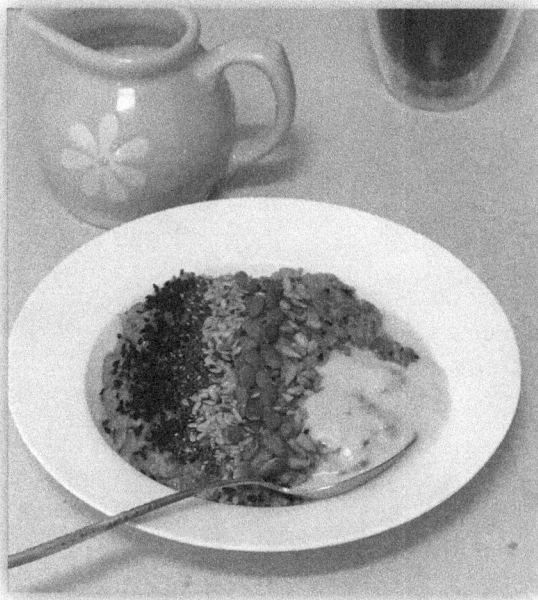

Ingredients

- ⅓ cup quinoa flakes
- ⅓ cup seeds (flaxseeds/ linseeds, chia, sesame, pepitas and sunflower seeds)
- Water or coconut milk (enough to cover ingredients)
- A dollop of coconut cream

Method

1. Add water or coconut milk and cook on a stove top till ready (stir frequently).

2. Serve with a dollop of coconut cream.

Fruit free Nut and Seed Muesli

Ingredients

- ¾ cup pecan nuts
- ½ cup macadamia nuts
- ½ cup walnuts
- ½ cup almonds
- ¼ cup pistachios
- 1 cup shredded coconut
- ½ cup pepitas
- ½ cup sunflower seeds
- ½ cup poppy seeds
- ½ cup chia seeds
- ½ cup sesame seeds
- ½ cup coconut oil

Suggestions

You can use this muesli for breakfast with almond or coconut milk, or add to salads, or even use to make protein balls for snacks.

Method

1. Preheat oven to 160°C /320°F.

2. Place all nuts in a processor and pulse a few times to mix and roughly chop.

3. Melt coconut oil.

4. Add the pepitas, sunflower seeds and coconut to the nut mix.

5. Pour in the oil and stir it through.

6. Spread out on a large oven tray lined with baking paper and put in the oven.

7. Cook for 10 minutes stirring the contents of the tray around a couple of times to make sure it doesn't burn but that all contents get a bit roasted.

8. Remove from oven and let cool.

9. Store in airtight jar in the fridge.

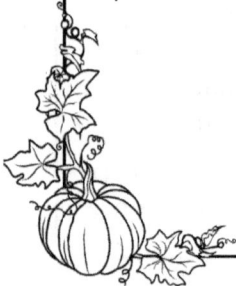

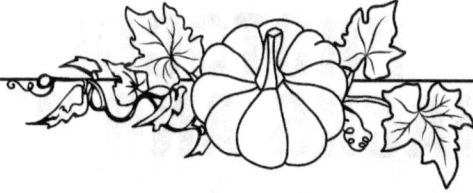

Chia Pudding with Protein Powder

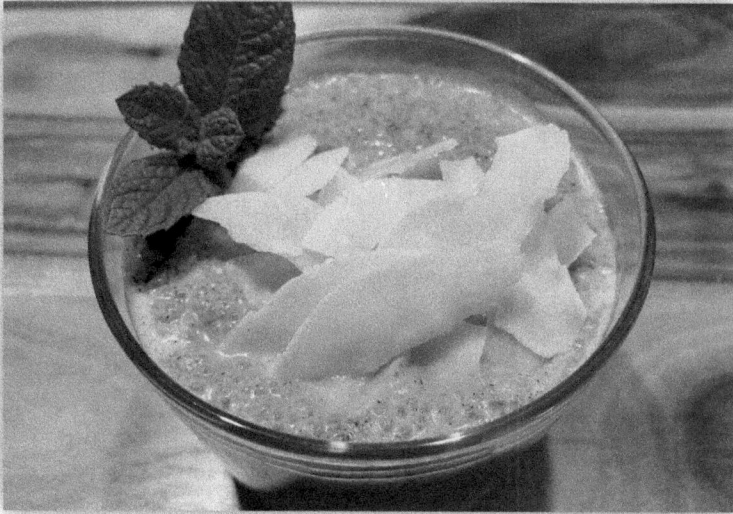

Ingredients

- ½ cup coconut milk (make sure sugars are under 6 per 100 grams)
- 1 teaspoon pure vanilla extract
- ¼ cup chia seeds
- 1 scoop of protein powder (make sure sugars are under 6 per 100 grams)
- ½ cup other milk of choice (rice or almond) (make sure sugars are under 6 per 100 grams)

Method

1. Mix all ingredients until well combined

2. Refrigerate until it sets (about an hour).

3. Enjoy!

MY FAVORITE PROTOCOL SNACKS AND DIPS

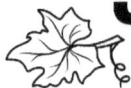

Protein Balls

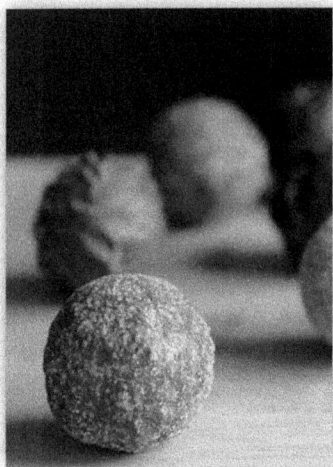

Ingredients

- 1-2 scoops Protein powder
- ½ cup melted Coconut oil
- ¼ cup Nut butter
- ¼ cup Flaxseed/linseed meal
- ¼ cup Almond meal
- ¼ cup Chia seeds
- Coconut for rolling
- 1 teaspoon Beetroot powder Optional

Method

1. Mix the ingredients together to right consistency to hold the shape.

2. Make into balls then roll in coconut and/or beetroot powder – there's no sugar added, but this is a yummy treat to look forward to. You can also add collagen powder to the balls too.

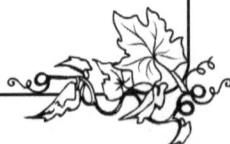

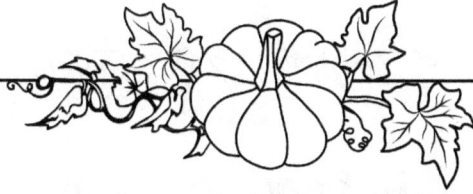

Fruit Free Muesli Balls

Refer to my fruit free breakfast muesli recipe and then make the muesli into balls to use as snacks too.

Other healthy protocol snack suggestions

- Boiled egg
- Carrot and celery sticks
- Vegetable dip – making your own is easy, then at least you know what is in it
- For more ideas get my recipe booklet at: www.karlenegeorgiadis.com.au/recipes

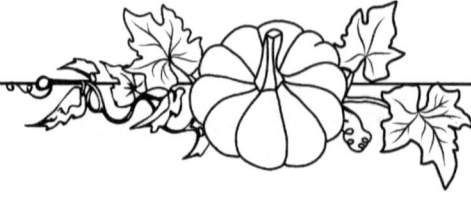

Nut and seed Dip

Building good bacteria takes consistent effort but it doesn't have to be boring OR flavorless.

This is an interesting dip to try to excite your taste buds, but it won't leave you feeling bloated or heavy afterwards.

Ingredients
- ½ cup raw cashews
- ⅛ cup of pine nuts
- 1 ½ tablespoons lemon juice
- 2 teaspoons of apple cider vinegar
- 1 cup of almond milk (read the label and check the sugar content), plus 1-3 more tablespoons
- ¼ cup of water
- ½ tsp Himalayan crystal salt
- ¼ teaspoon of crushed yellow mustard
- 1 tablespoon of gluten free corn flour or arrowroot or tapioca flour
- ½ teaspoon paprika
- ⅛ teaspoon turmeric

Method
1. Mix and blend all the ingredients and add to a small saucepan.
2. Heat slowly on the stove top and be careful not to burn, stirring gently and until it thickens.
3. Add more almond milk if it needs to be thinned to get the right consistency.

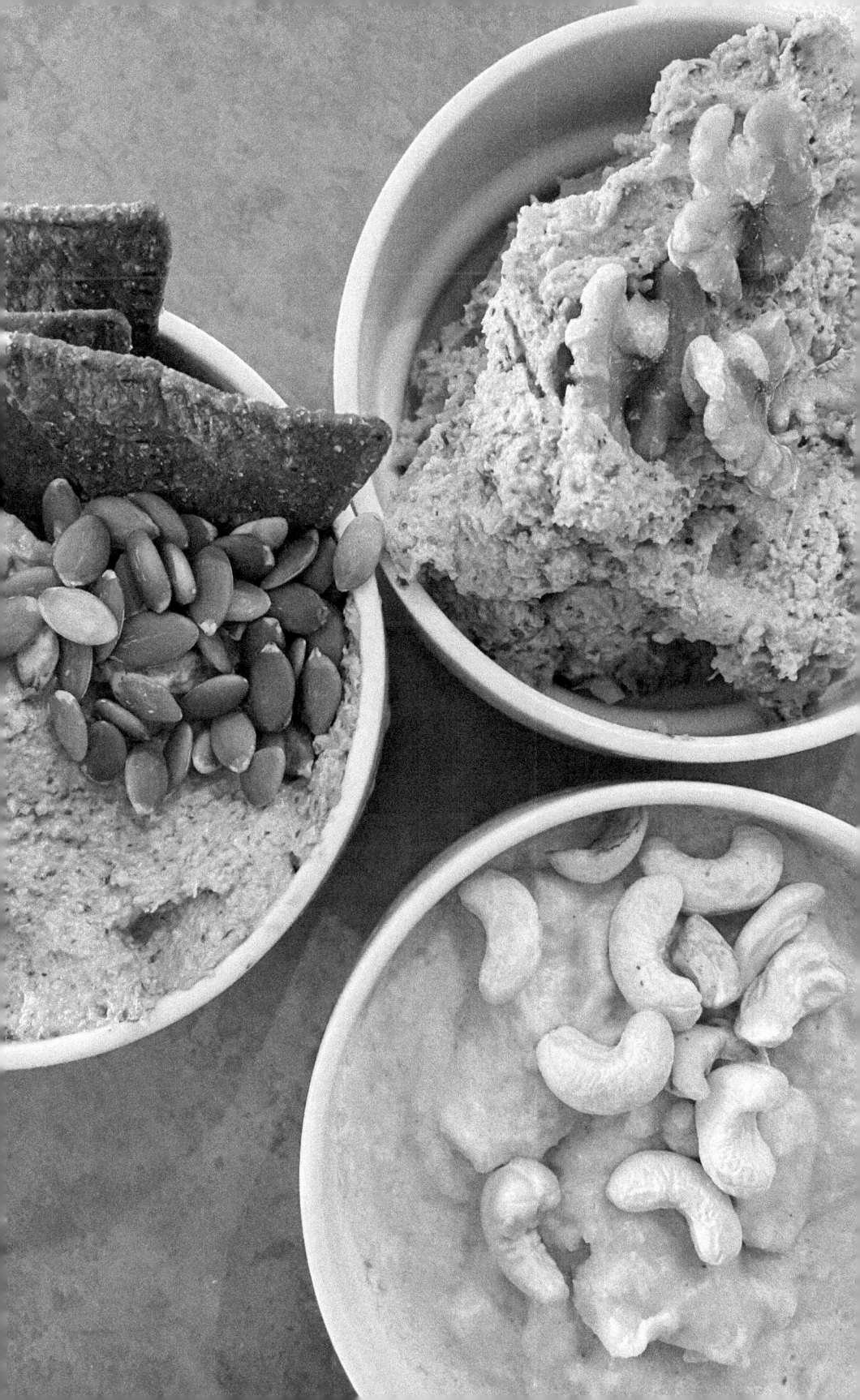

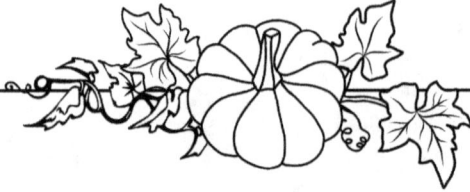

Roasted Pumpkin Dip

Pumpkin is your best friend when it comes to avoiding bloating and this dip can accompany a myriad of dishes. I add a spoonful on anything and everything.

Ingredients

- 500gms of butternut pumpkin cut into small chunks
- 3 tablespoons olive oil
- ½ cup of walnuts
- 2-4 teaspoons of cumin seeds depending on how much flavour you like
- ¼ cup of fresh coriander or more
- Sprinkle of nutmeg
- Salt and pepper to taste

Method

1. Roast the pumpkin in the oven at 180°C/360° Fcovered in oil and cook until tender to skewer.

2. Wait 10 minutes to cool.

3. Then blend all the ingredients together.

This dip provides yummy, sweet goodness without the sugar.

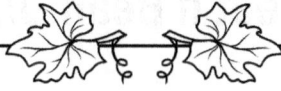

Zucchini Humus Dip

I often need a recipe for patients who need to build their bacteria, which is free from beans/legumes.

Leaving out beans/legumes in these cases is crucial.
You can also leave out the garlic if you know you don't tolerate it, OR maybe try roasting it a bit first – sometimes people tolerate garlic cooked, but not raw.

Have a play with this lovely Bacteroides-building high-zinc recipe.

Ingredients

- 2 cups of raw zucchini chopped into small chunks
- 1 ½ cups of pepitas
- ½ cup unhulled tahini
- 2 tablespoons lemon juice
- 3 tablespoons olive oil
- ¼ cup basil leaves
- 1-2 small cloves of garlic – roasted if needed (optional)
- 1 teaspoon of cracked pepper
- Salt to taste

Method

Blend this green goodness until smooth. Just put it all into the blender and whizz.

Serve with a few pepitas sprinkled on top.

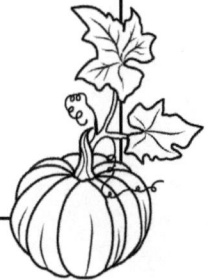

Beet n Bean Dip

Ingredients

- 4 small beetroots cooked and peeled
- ½ can cannellini beans
- 2 tablespoons fennel seeds
- 1 lemon squeezed
- 2 tablespoons of olive oil
- Generous salt to taste
- Generous pepper to taste
- Sprig of fresh dill – as much as you like/to taste

Method

1. In a blender buzz all ingredients to the right consistency and add a sprig of dill on top to serve.

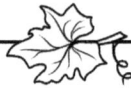

LUNCH IDEAS AND SOUPS

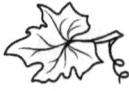

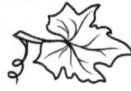

Be Free Wrap
(use a multi grain or sweet potato wrap)

- Add salad of choice (make it colourful)
- Avocado
- Alfalfa

- If you are ok with cooked chicken add that – or cooked lamb or beef

Pea and Hemp Burgers

Vegan-friendly, enjoy with salad. (Refer to my dinners on a protocol for my pea and hemp burger recipe.)

- For variety in a salad, sprinkle my Fruit Free Muesli over the salad or in your wrap. Refer also to the recipe in the breakfast section of my recipe booklet.

Vegetable Frittata Slice

Download recipe in my free recipe booklet: www.book.karlene.com.au/recipes

Soup of choice using a bone broth base

- Add protein of choice and plenty of vegetables to your bone broth

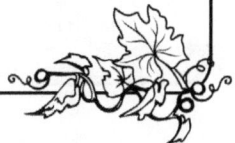

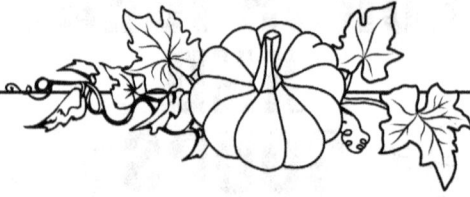

Bone Broth

(this is the base recipe from which all other soups can be built)

Ingredients

- 2kg organic chicken carcasses, or 2kgs of beef or lamb bones
- Cold filtered water to cover, plus extra water to add during cooking
- Dash of apple cider vinegar

Method

1. For red meat bones, bake for 20 minutes in the oven before making this broth.
2. Cover the bones well in water in a slow cooker or large saucepan.
3. Add a dash of apple cider vinegar.
4. Bring to boil and skim off fat and froth from top.
5. Turn down to a very gentle simmer (just so the water is moving.)
   a. For three-four hours (saucepan.)
   b. For six-seven hours (slow cooker.)
   c. Keep the lid on but top up with extra water when needed.
6. Leave to cool, strain and remove bones.
7. Place liquid in fridge overnight.
8. Next day, pour into jars and put in freezer.
9. The broth can be frozen for up to 3 months or kept in fridge for 5-7 days.

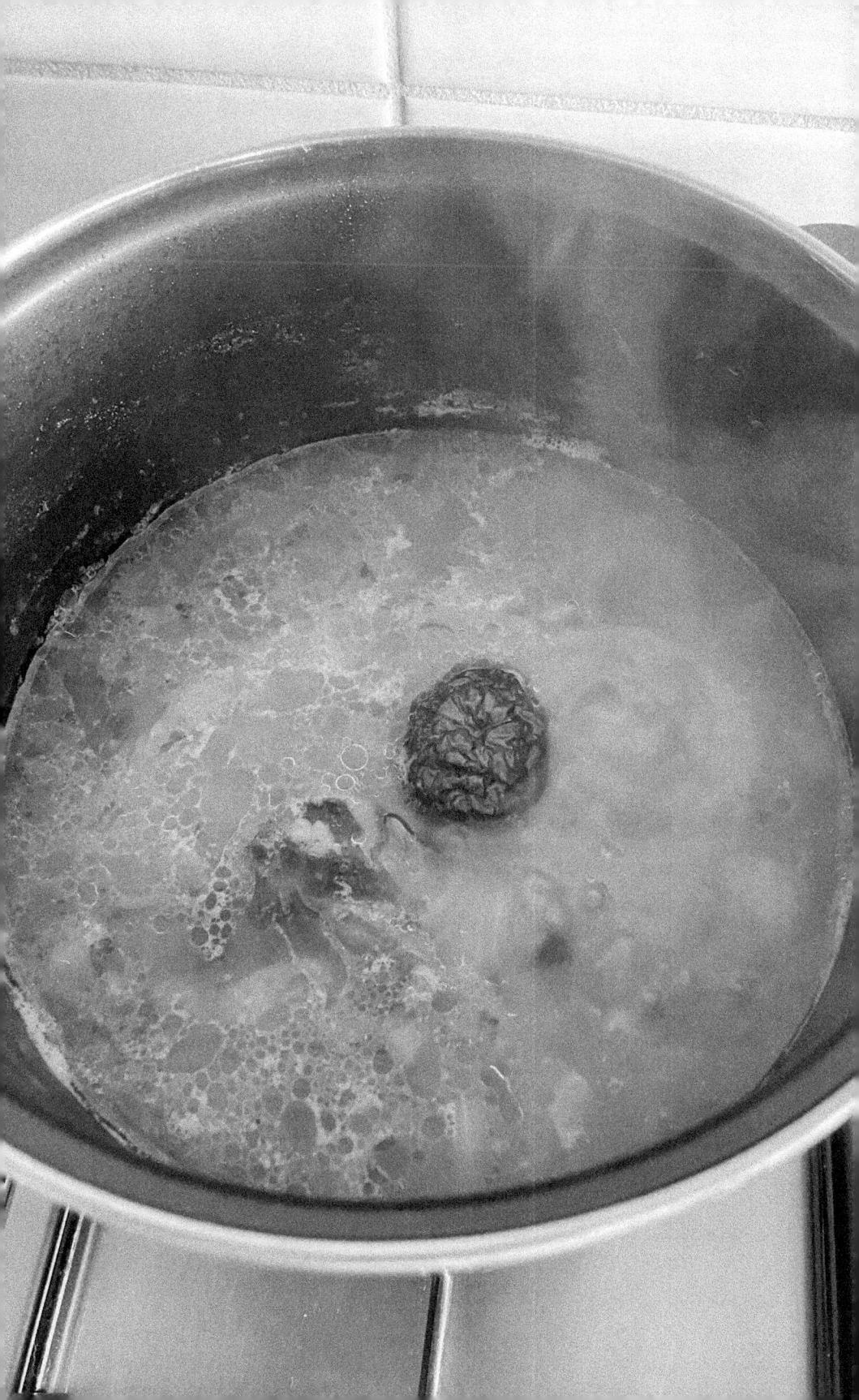

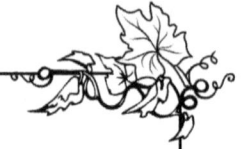

Chicken Noodle Soup

This is a well-known soup in my house for anything that ails you. I've adapted my protocol version from a recipe by Jude Blereau called *"Chicken soup to cure all ills."*

Ingredients

- 1 tablespoon virgin coconut oil
- 1 small leek, washed and thinly sliced
- 2 garlic cloves finely chopped (leave out if you are unable to have garlic)
- 2 celery stalks finely chopped
- 1 carrot finely diced
- 1 teaspoon fresh thyme leaves
- 1 teaspoon fresh sage leaves
- 1 large shiitake mushroom, quartered
- 1 litre of chicken stock
- 1 chicken leg
- 1 teaspoon dulse flakes
- 40gms peas
- 4-5 dark green leaves (collard greens, Tuscan kale or cos lettuce are ideal)
- 50 gms pasta (gluten free)
- 1 tablespoon finely chopped flat leaf parsley

Method

1. Place oil in large pot over medium heat.

2. Add leek, garlic, celery, carrot, and herbs and cook stirring frequently.

3. Add mushroom, chicken leg and stock and cover with lid and bring to boil.

4. Reduce to low heat and simmer for one hour.

5. Add dulse flakes, peas and greens, plus pasta and cook for another 10 minutes or until pasta is cooked. You can remove the chicken leg and strip the meat – returning the meat to the soup.

6. Adjust taste with salt and pepper.

7. Add parsley just before serving.

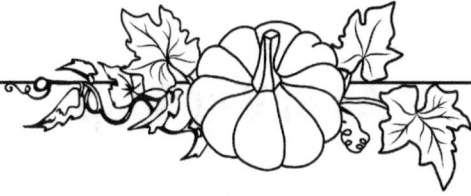

Pumpkin, Sweet Potato and Leek Soup

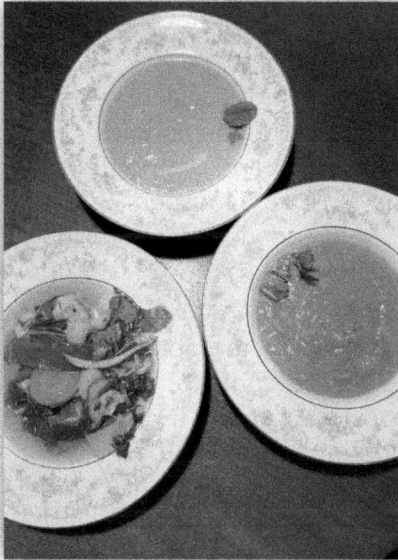

Ingredients

- 2 leeks thinly sliced
- ¼ Jap pumpkin diced (wash and leave the skin on)
- 1 medium sweet potato diced (washed and skin on)
- 1 litre of beef or chicken stock
- 400gm can of coconut milk
- Salt and pepper to taste
- Chopped mint for garnish

Method

1. Place all the ingredients in a pot with stock and cook until tender.

2. Blend or mash when cooked.

3. Add coconut milk and stir through.

4. Add salt and pepper to taste, heat through and serve.

5. Add chopped mint to garnish.

All in Veg Soup

Ingredients

- 2 leeks thinly sliced
- ½ swede
- 1 carrot
- 3 bok choy
- 2 cloves garlic
- Handful of beans
- Handful of snow peas
- Handful of sugar snap peas
- Fresh coriander chopped or parsley if preferred
- 3 peppercorns
- 1 bay leaf
- ¼ head of cauliflower
- ½ head broccoli
- 2 stalks of celery
- 1 litre of lamb or chicken stock
- 2 cups zucchini noodles or konjac noodles
- Salt and pepper to taste
- Extra chopped coriander for garnish

Method

Place the harder dense vegetables in the pot with the garlic, bay leaf and peppercorns to cook a bit before adding the softer green veggies so they are just cooked through by the time it is ready to consume.

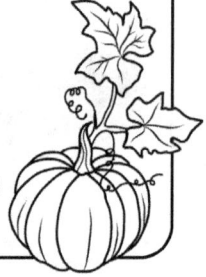

Fennel and Pea Soup

Ingredients

- 1 fennel bulb chopped
- 2 cups of peas
- 1 clove of garlic
- 1 tin of coconut milk
- 1 ½ litres of chicken or lamb stock

Method

Place chopped fennel and peas in pot with garlic and stock. Cook until tender.

Blend ingredients and then add coconut milk. Heat through before serving.

Garnish with fresh chopped mint.

DINNER IDEAS

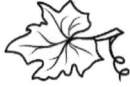

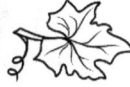

- Meat of choice and vegetables or salad (or both) cooked your way
- Smaller fish are great (whiting, dory, garfish, flathead tails etc.)
- Stir fry with a small amount of brown rice or quinoa or use a blend of these
- Or try brown rice noodles or the slimmer noodles made from konjac root

Vegetable Frittata Slice

Suitable for breakfast, lunch or dinner.

Ingredients

- 6 eggs
- 1 zucchini grated
- 1 carrot grated
- 3 tablespoons of chopped fresh herbs (I like coriander but parsley, basil, dill would all work too)
- ¼ cup coconut oil
- ¼ cup almond flour (or gluten free corn flour/ coconut flour/green banana flour)

Be adventurous with your vegetable choice, this is great for any vegetables that you have waiting in the crisper, I used corn in my last batch.

Method

1. Preheat oven to 180°C /360°F.
2. Blend or finely chop vegetables and herbs and add to a large bowl.
3. Whisk eggs and add to the bowl.
4. Add oil and flour.
5. Stir well and season to taste.
6. Pour into a greased quiche tin or pan and pop in the oven for 20 to 30 minutes or until cooked throughout.
7. Allow to cool before slicing.

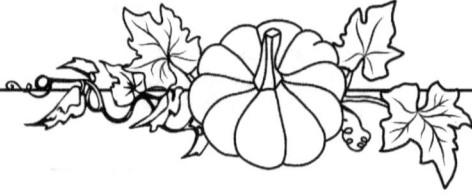

Pea and Hemp Burgers

These are vegan-friendly and suitable for lunch or dinners.

Ingredients

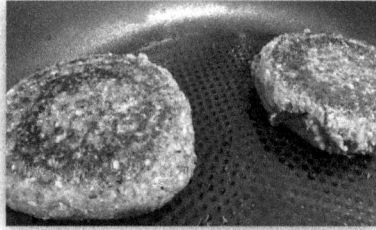

- 500gm peas cooked, strained then blitzed (making them quite fluffy and mushy)
- 2 large handfuls of coriander or any green herb finely chopped
- ½ cup of hemp seeds
- ¼ cup corn flour, or any other flour you prefer to use
- ¼ cup rice crumbs
- Salt & pepper to taste

Though I haven't added garlic or onions, you could add these of course which would enhance the flavor and goodness.

Method

1. Mush the peas and all ingredients together and form into patties.
2. Shallow fry in coconut oil until golden on each side and warmed through.

* I use the burgers for either lunch or dinner. For lunch, I use these as the base for a very colourful wrap. I add pesto and a tahini mayonnaise, a handful of greens and some grated carrot. YUM!

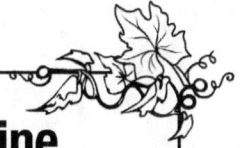

No Tomato – Low Histamine Spag Sauce

This is not the prettiest sauce I've ever seen, but when looking for a low histamine solution this is a great option.

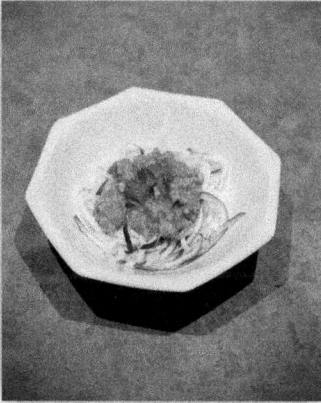

Ingredients

- 3 zucchinis
- 3 carrots
- ½ onion
- 1 clove garlic
- Handful of coriander or parsley
- 1 liter bone broth stock
- Olive oil
- Salt and pepper to taste
- 500gm mince of choice – veal is great for soft flavor

Method

1. Chop and quarter the zucchini and carrot and place in a steamer to cook until tender. Then place in a blender and blitz – this is now your sauce.
2. Prepare the onion and garlic and fry in a bit of olive oil.
3. Add the mince and brown it well – until it smells roasted.
4. Then add the sauce you prepared earlier and the stock liquid.
5. Adjust taste with salt and pepper.
6. Chop through parsley or coriander before serving.

I serve this on zucchini noodles or konjac noodles. It's a winner!!

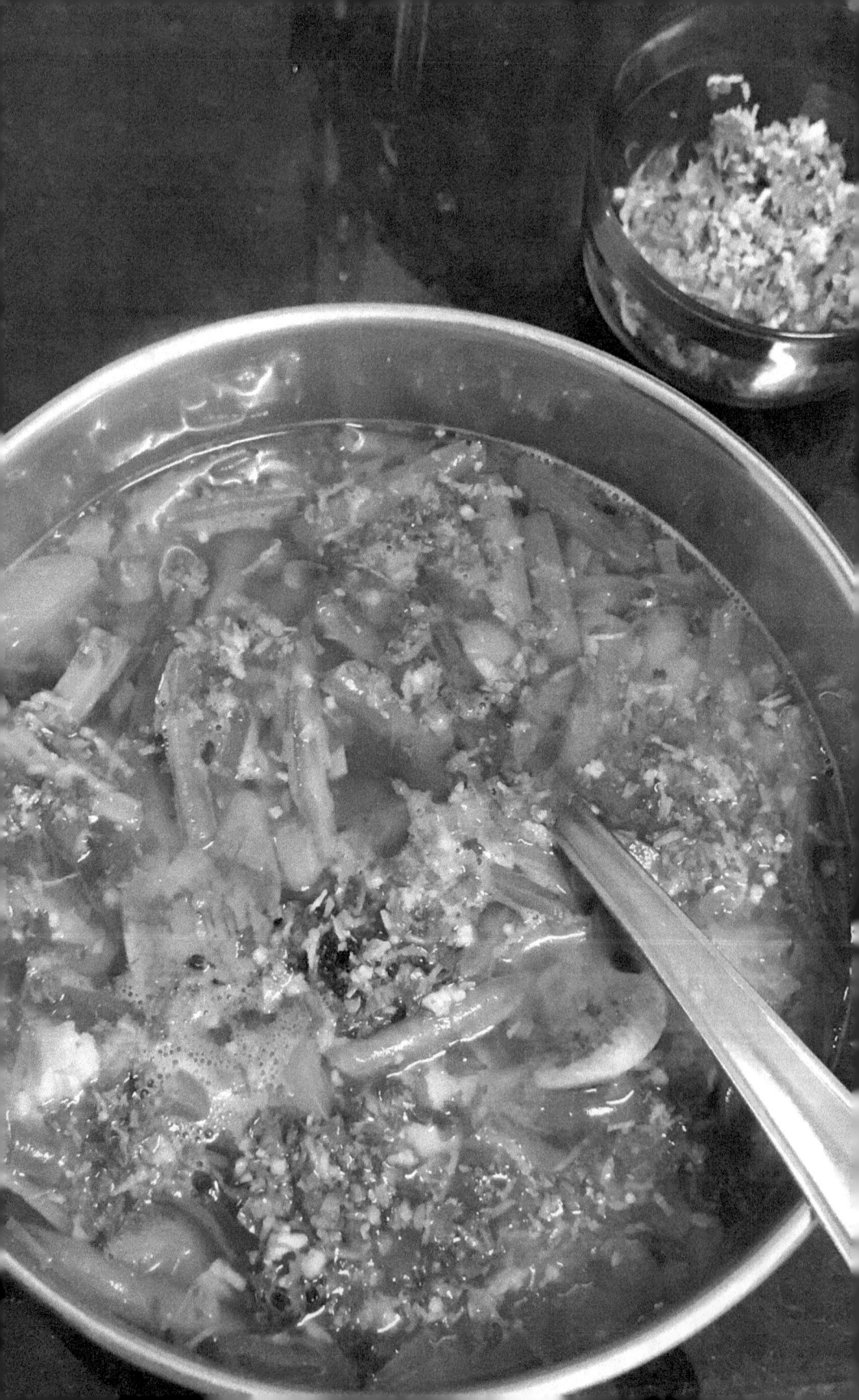

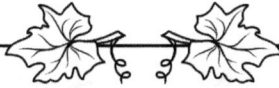

Osso Bucco

This is not traditional; it's my idea of a one pot wonder, slow cooked and using meat on bones and with loads of vegetables.

Ingredients

- 2 beef osso bucco shin pieces
- 2 sticks of celery
- 2 carrots chopped
- 1 leek
- Cauliflower – about 3 florets
- Broccoli
- Beans (de-strung)
- 1 onion (chopped)
- 2 cloves garlic
- Dash of apple cider vinegar
- 6 peppercorns
- 1 bay leaf
- Salt
- Water to cover

Method

1. Sear the shin bones in a splash of olive oil and then place in the slow cooker
2. Cover with the vegetables and all other ingredients
3. Cover with water.
4. Slow cook for 6 hours.
5. Serve with fresh gremolata if this is to your liking.

Gremolata

- 1 lemon (rind grated)
- 1 clove of crushed garlic
- Handful of parsley

Top your osso bucco with gremolata before serving.

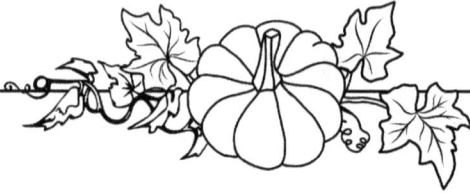

Ox Tail Casserole

Have you ever bought ox (cow) tail before? This is definitely one to ask your butcher for as it has so much bone and cartilage goodness. Here is my standard soup/casserole recipe for you to play with the next time you order your oxtail.

Ingredients

- 2.5kg ox tail
- Olive oil
- 2 leeks
- 4 carrots
- 2 stalks of celery
- Sprig each of thyme and sage
- 4 fresh bay leaves
- 4 cloves
- 6 peppercorns
- Beef stock
- Dash of apple cider vinegar

Method

1. Roast the tails first in the oven (this improves the flavour) at 200°C/390°F for 20 minutes.

2. Prepare all vegetables.

3. Add all everything to the slow cooker and cook on high for four-five hours.

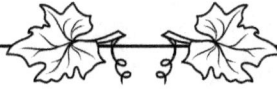

Lamb Shank Stew

Another amazing bone and meat broth to serve your gut health well.

Ingredients

- 2 lamb shanks
- 3 stalks of celery
- 1 leek
- 3 carrots
- Onion
- Parsnip
- Swede
- 1 clove garlic
- Peppercorns
- Himalayan crystal salt to taste
- Sprig of rosemary, thyme and sage
- ½ cup brown rice/black rice/wild rice
- Dash of apple cider vinegar
- Water to cover plus more added as it evaporates

Method

1. No browning or pre-baking required.

2. Place all ingredients in a pot and simmer for three-four hours.

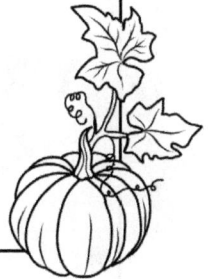

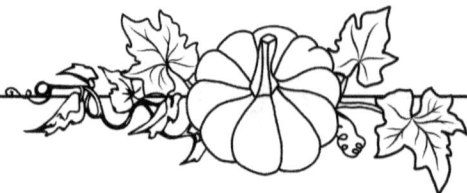

Lamb Necks

There are so many beautiful parts of the animal that we don't think to cook, but they are nutrient rich and healing for the gut.

Ingredients

- 4 x 450gm lamb necks
- 2 onions
- 2 sprigs rosemary
- 8 sprigs thyme
- 1 fennel bulb sliced
- 4 carrots
- Dash of apple cider vinegar
- Flat parsley to serve and a squeeze of lemon
- Quinoa or sweet potato and pumpkin mash to serve

Method

1. Brown the necks in a pan with a bit of olive oil before putting them in the slow cooker.

2. Add all other ingredients except the parsley and squeeze of lemon.

3. Cook on high for four-five hours or low for seven-eight hours.

4. Serve with splash or parsley and squeeze of lemon.

5. Serve on quinoa or sweet potato and pumpkin mash.

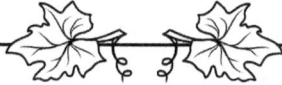

Chicken Slow Cook Casserole

Purchase skinless chicken thighs on the bone for this recipe. This is a slow cooker recipe but can be adapted to go in the oven in a casserole, or in a pressure cooker.

Ingredients

- 6 skinless chicken thighs (with bone still in)
- 2 teaspoons apple cider vinegar
- 1 teaspoon olive oil
- 1 onion chopped
- 2 stalks of celery
- 1 medium leek thinly slices
- 3 medium carrots chopped
- 1 clove garlic
- 2 capsicums sliced into strips
- 1 teaspoon of fresh or dried oregano
- 2 cups of chicken stock
- 1 swede roughly chopped
- 200gm button mushrooms sliced
- ½ lemon juice
- 1 handful of fresh chopped parsley

Method

1. Heat the oil in a heavy pan and brown the chicken thighs for approximately three minutes then add these to the slow cooker.

2. In the same pan add the onions, garlic and all the vegetables, sauté with apple cider vinegar then add to the slow cooker.

3. Add everything else except the mushrooms, lemon juice and parsley.

4. Cook in the slow cooker for three-four hours on high (six-seven hours on low).

5. Add the mushrooms in the last 30 minutes.

6. Serve with the lemon squeezed on top and sprinkle chopped parsley.

Chicken Korma

This is a lovely rich curry dish with the added value of coconut milk and the nutrient goodness of bones.

Ingredients

- 6 skinless chicken thighs on the bone
- Olive oil
- 400ml coconut milk
- 1 teaspoon ginger
- 2 tablespoons almond meal (or collagen powder)
- Flaked almonds toasted
- Coriander sprigs
- Cooked brown rice or quinoa to serve

The Korma Curry Paste

- 2 onions
- 4 cloves garlic
- 2 teaspoon turmeric
- 2 teaspoons garam masala
- 1 teaspoon ground coriander
- ½ teaspoon ground cumin
- ½ teaspoon paprika
- ¼ teaspoon ground cardamom
- Pinch of nutmeg
- Pinch chilli flakes

Vegetables

Combination of chopped pieces of:

- Sweet potato
- Pumpkin
- Cauliflower
- Carrot

Method

1. To make the curry paste place all the curry ingredients into a blender and whizz.

2. Add oil to a heavy pan and add the curry paste and let it heat and fill the room with its aroma.

3. Add the chicken thighs to the pan and coat with the curry paste.

4. Add the milk, ginger and almond meal or collagen powder.

5. Add chopped vegetables and cook slowly for three-four hours.

6. Serve with toasted almonds and chopped coriander, cooked brown rice or quinoa.

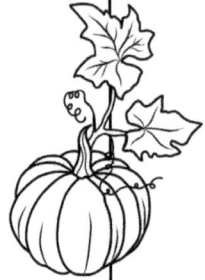

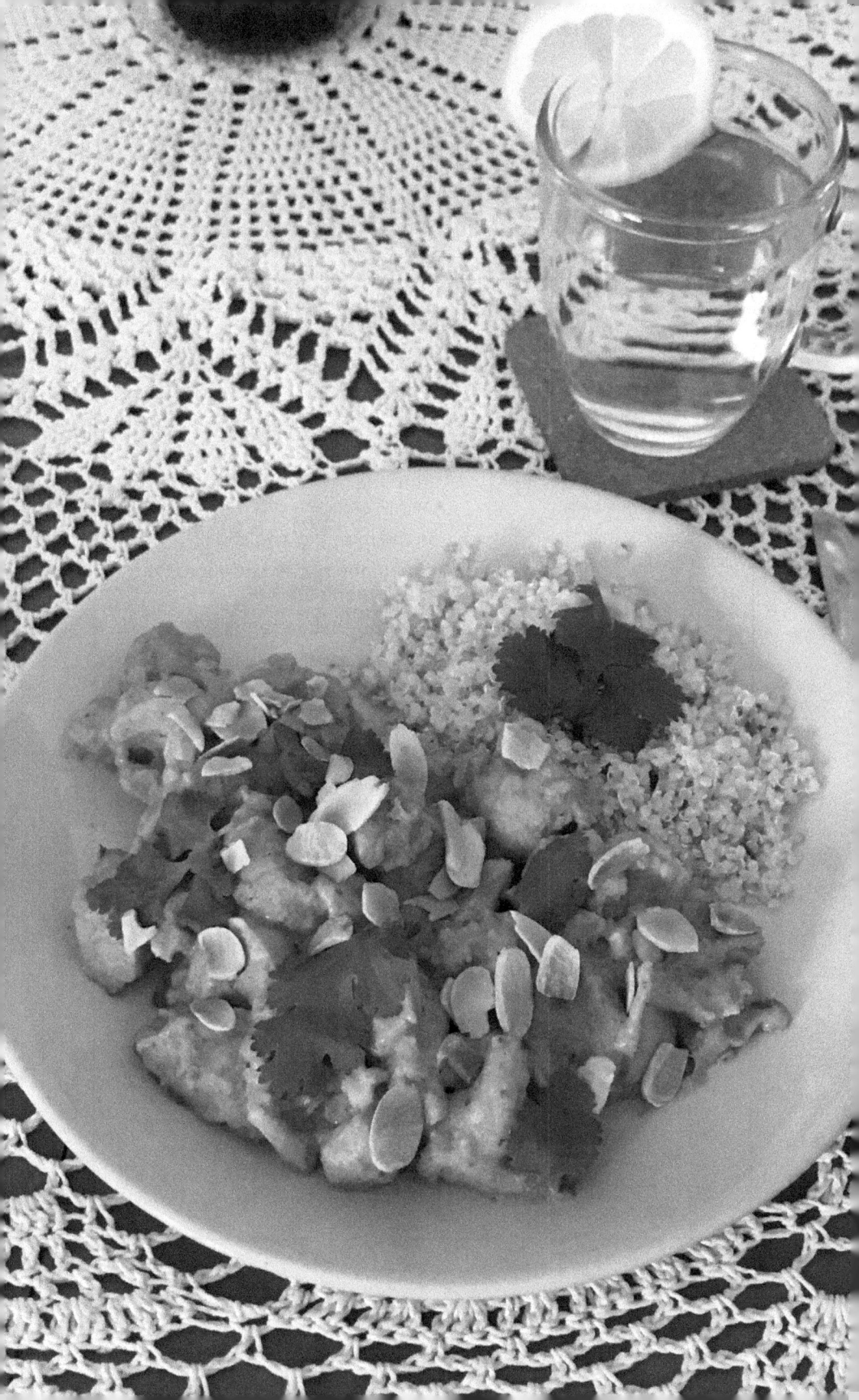

CAKES, SLICES AND CHRISTMAS CHEER

Sago Plum Pudding

This is my mother's original recipe with tweaks by me to make it more gut friendly.

Ingredients

- 4 tablespoons of sago or tapioca balls
- 1 cup of milk almond milk or coconut milk
- 1 ½ teaspoons bicarb get the aluminium-free type from the health food store
- 2 tablespoons butter or coconut oil
- ¾ cup brown sugar (omit if wanting to be sugar free, use less or none at all)
- ½ teaspoon grated lemon rind
- 1 cup soft white breadcrumbs (gluten free)
- 1 cup mixed dried fruit my mother always threw in figs, dates and raisins and red glace cherries for the Christmas look but not the green ones (not sure why) and then she added slivered almonds for crunch
- Pinch of Himalayan crystal salt

Method

1. Pour the milk on the washed sago and soak overnight.
2. In the morning add soda.
3. Cream the butter and sugar then add lemon rind.
4. Add the soaked sago.
5. Fold in breadcrumbs.
6. Add fruit, salt and mix it really well.
7. Turn into a well-greased over-proof bowl or dish.
8. Cover with grease-proof paper, then cover with foil over top.
9. Steam bowl in a large pot with water for two and a half to three hours. Remember to check the water level regularly and top up as needed. Boil any additional water in the jug first to keep the simmer going.
10. Turn out carefully (take care to ensure it comes out in one piece. This was always such a special moment at home, my mother would be very happy when the pudding came out in one piece, but it always tasted so good any which way it came out.

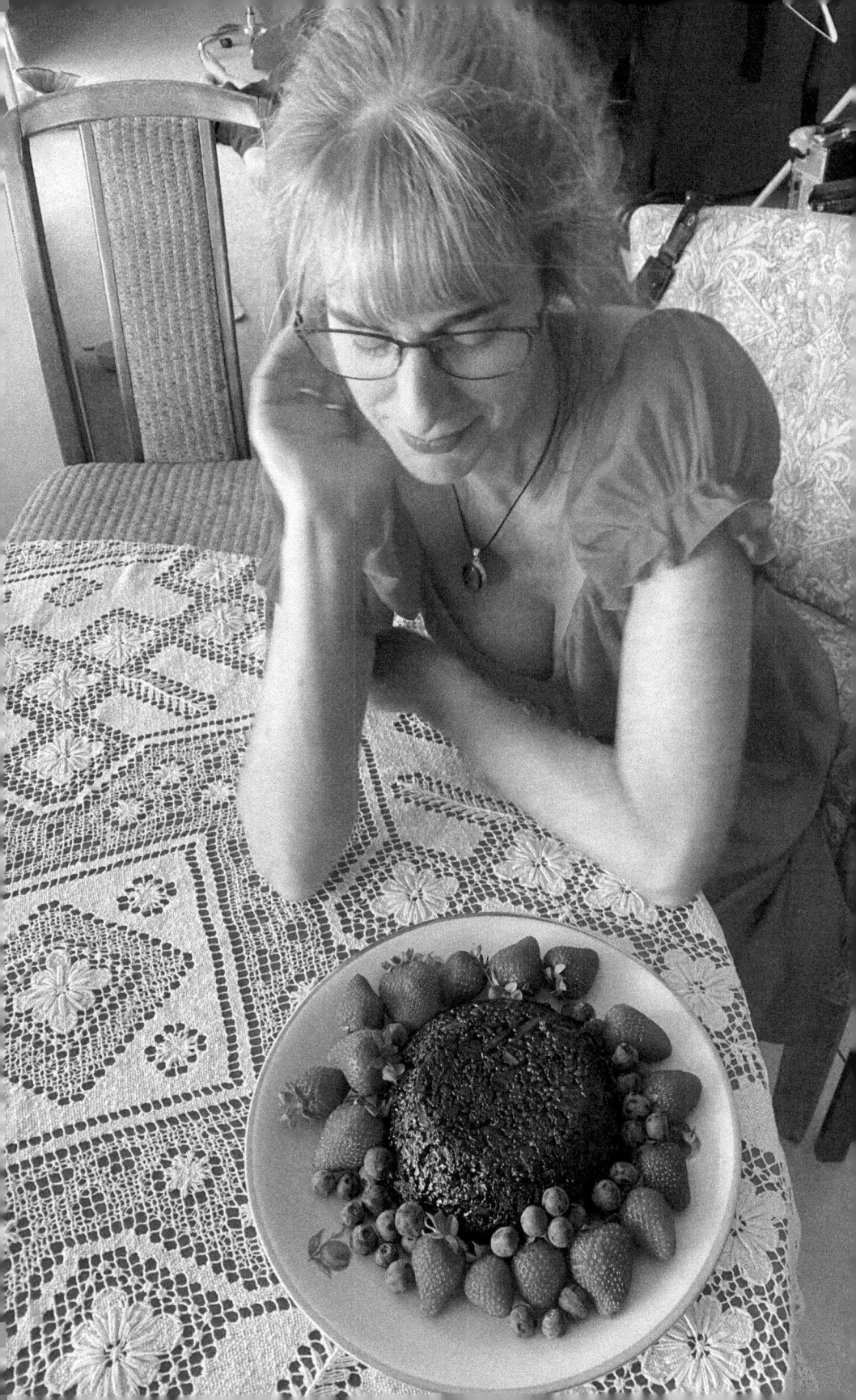

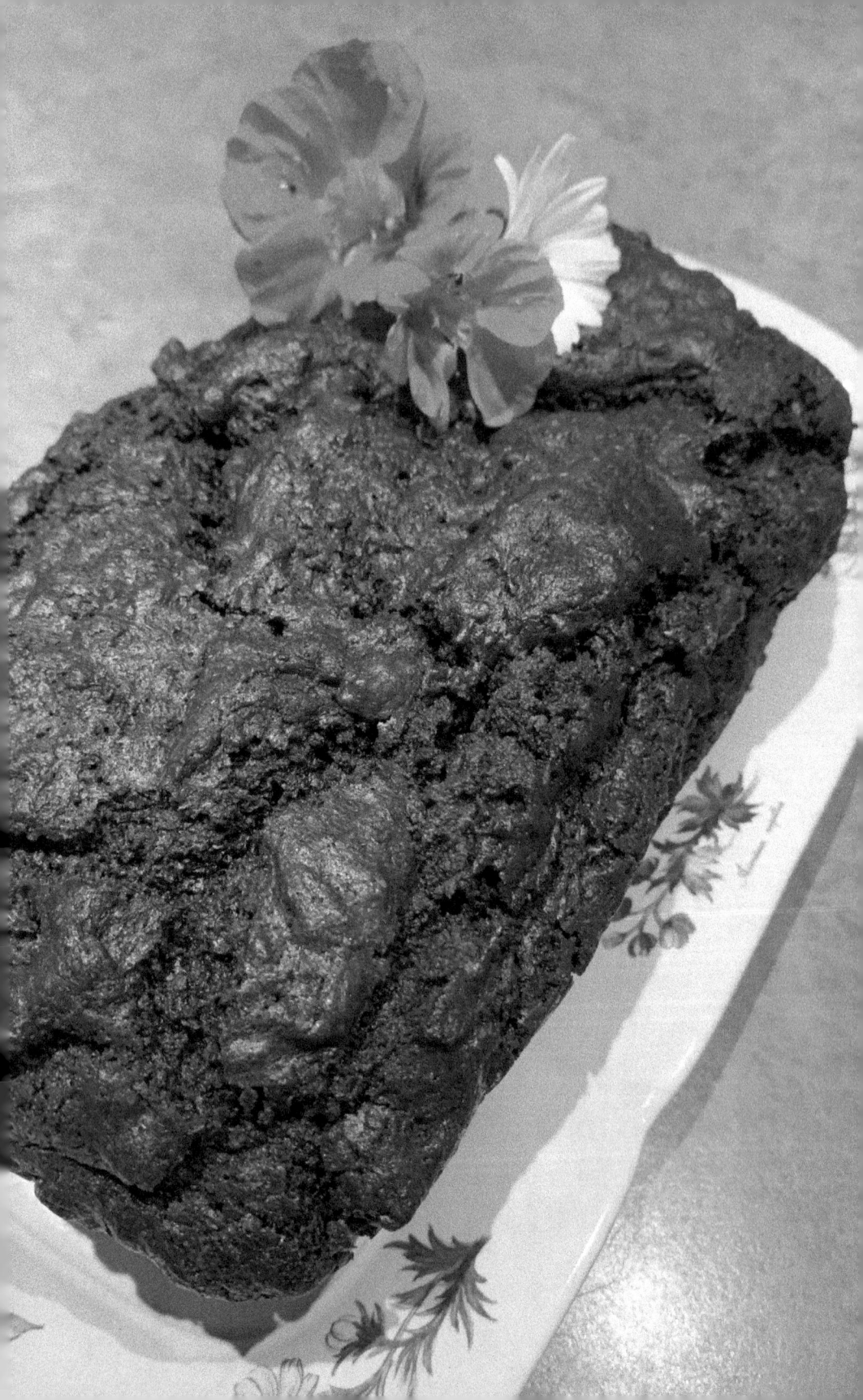

Chocolate Beetroot Cake – Jacked-Up

I've spent time adapting my signature chocolate beetroot cake. I've made it even better using homegrown beetroot and adding powdered bilberry. The bilberry is pure genius! It is not only yummy, but good for your immunity too.

Ingredients

- 1 ½ cups cacao
- 2 cups gluten free flour
- 2 teaspoons baking powder
- 1 teaspoon bicarb soda
- 1 ½ cups coconut sugar
- 1 cup coconut oil, or 1 cup macadamia oil, whichever you prefer
- 2 teaspoons vanilla essence
- ¼ teaspoon ground cardamom
- 6 eggs
- 2 large beetroots
- ¼ cup of dry ground bilberry

Method

1. Boil unpeeled beetroot. Once the beetroot is cooked, let it cool and then peel it. I usually cook the beetroot the day before I make the cake. This way there are no burnt fingers in the peeling process.
2. Preheat oven to 170°C /340°F.
3. Grease and paper a springform pan. The recipe will make either a 24cm round cake, or a 20cm round cake, or 12 large muffins.
4. Chop the beetroot up and blend in a food processor.
5. Use 1 ½ cups of the pureed beetroot for the base of the cake batter. Sift together cocoa, flour, baking powder, bicarb soda into the batter.
6. Beat the eggs.
7. Add the oil to the beaten eggs and mix well into the batter.
8. Add the sugar and vanilla essence. Mix well.
9. Pour into the baking pan and bake for approximately 50 minutes.

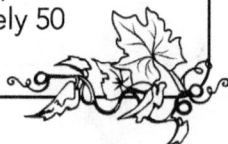

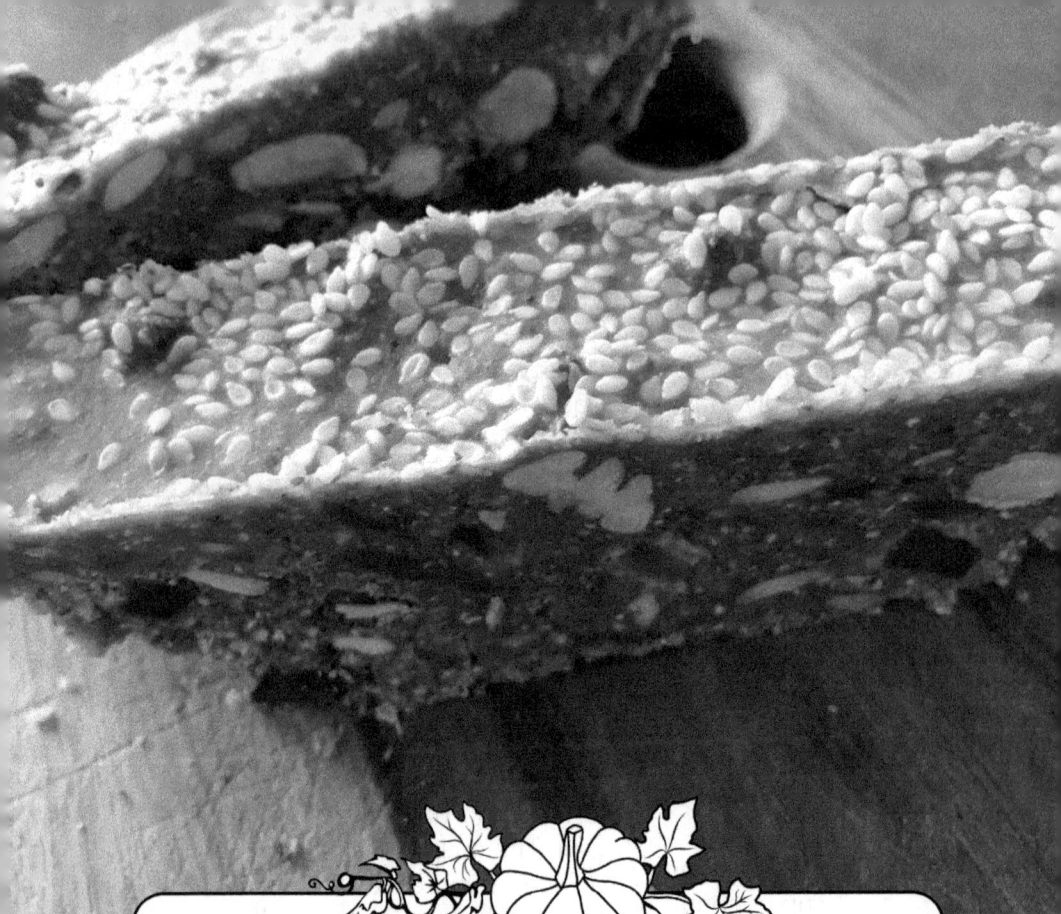

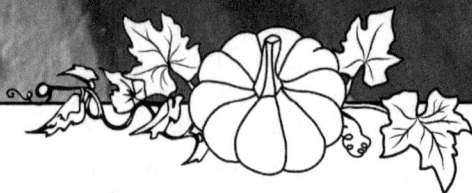

Satisfaction Slice

This slice is a way to trick the taste buds into thinking they're getting a sweet treat, when really, we are just loading up on brain food.

Heads up, these are not sweet! They seem to be sweet, and the look, texture and smell all say yummy this is sweet. But in actual fact there is very little sweetness. Instead, there is a heap of nutrition…brain food and good ol' satisfaction.

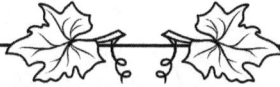

Ingredients

- ½ cup coconut oil melted
- 100gm cacao butter melted
- ½ cup linseed (flaxseed), sunflower seed and almond (LSA) meal
- ½ cup almond meal
- ¼ cup pepitas crushed/blitzed
- ¼ cup walnuts crushed/blitzed
- ¼ cup of nut butter, such as almond, cashew and brazil (ABC) nut spread
- ¼ cup chia seeds
- 1 vanilla pod
- 1 tablespoon cacao powder
- 2 tablespoons naked ginger pieces finely chopped
- Sometimes I throw in whole nuts

Method

1. Melt the oil and cacao butter in a small saucepan.

2. Place all the dry ingredients in a bowl.

3. Mix in nut butter and melted oil and butter mix.

4. Press into a lined casserole dish or loaf pan.

5. Sprinkle the top with sesame seeds or crushed pepitas or coconut flakes.

6. Set in the fridge.

7. Once it sets remove from the dish and cut into slices with a sharp knife.

8. After slicing mine into portions, I wrap them in grease proof paper.

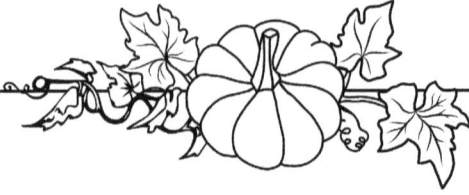

Five Seed Crackers

Thank you to Erica for sharing this recipe with me!

Ingredients

- 1 cup sunflower seeds
- ¾ cup pepitas
- ½ cup chia seeds
- 1 teaspoon Himalayan crystal salt
- ¼ cup flaxseeds/linseeds
- ¼ cup sesame seeds
- 1 ½ cups water
- 1 teaspoon dried herbs

Method

1. Pre-heat oven to 170°C /340°F.
2. Mix all ingredients and leave for 15 minutes.
3. Stir well.
4. Use two baking trays.
5. Smooth mixture across the two baking trays about 3-4 mm thick.
6. Bake for 50 minutes or until brown and crisp. May need extra time.
7. Allow to cool and break up into bite size pieces.

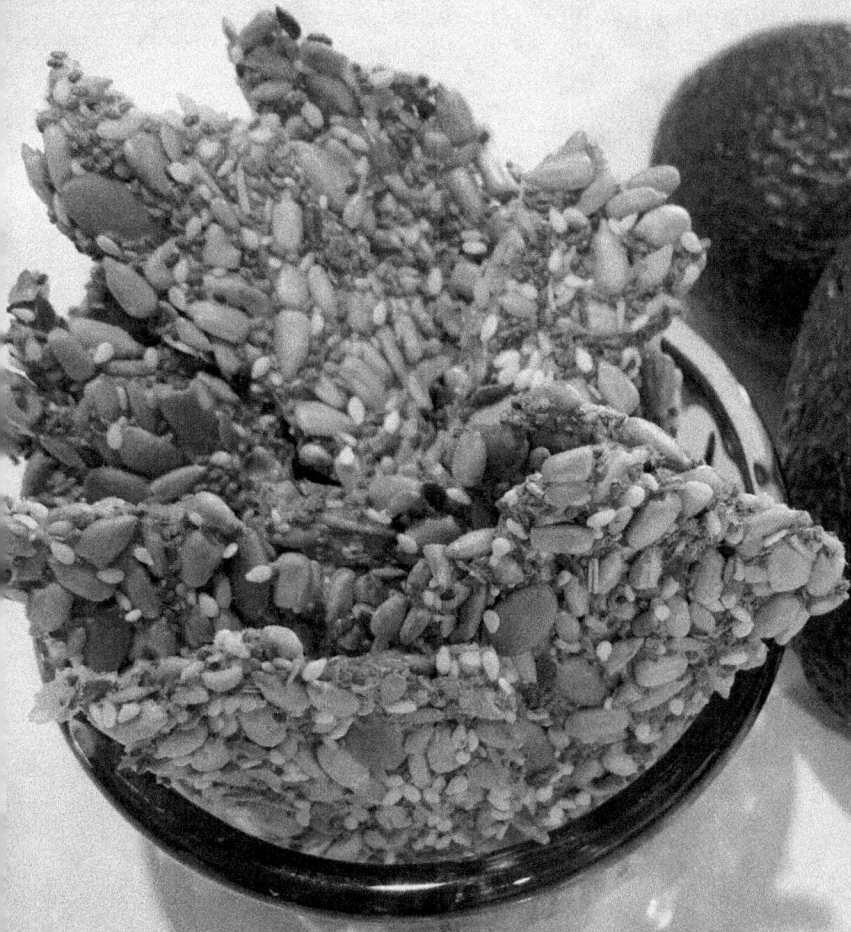

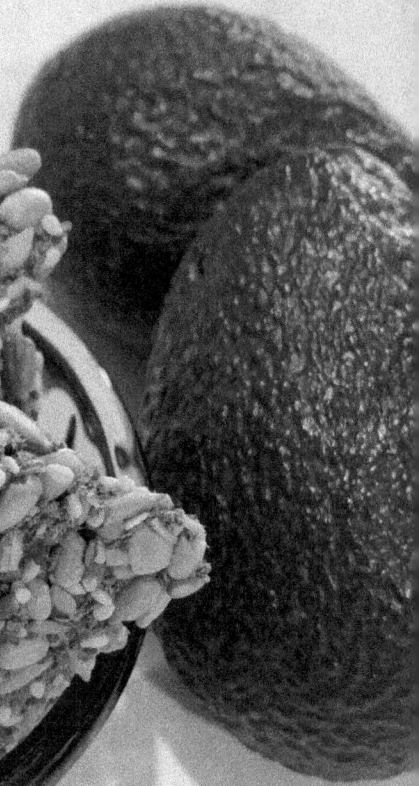

FREE RECIPE BOOKLET

For more recipes including further salads, smoothies, snacks, lunches and dinners download the complete recipe booklet with many more suggestions here: www.book.karlene.com.au/recipes

Flow slice

This slice is a powerful anti-inflammatory and very yummy recipe.

Ingredients Bottom Layer

- ½ cup ground almonds
- ½ cup flaxseeds/linseeds, sunflower seeds and almond (LSA) meal
- 2 tablespoons of coconut oil
- 2 tablespoons of tahini (unhulled is best)
- 1 tablespoon of maple syrup (or use equivalent of stevia, but no inulin if you are on a protocol)
- 1 teaspoon ground turmeric
- ½ teaspoon dry ginger

Ingredients Top Layer

- 1 tablespoon coconut oil
- 4 tablespoons of nut butter (I use almond)
- 1 tablespoon of sweetener (I use maple syrup but stevia or rice malt syrup would work)
- 1 cm grated fresh ginger
- Juice from ½ a lemon
- Sprinkles of shredded coconut

Method Bottom Layer

1. To make the base, line a 20cm x 10cm loaf pan with cooking paper.
2. Melt the coconut oil and mix all the ingredients together well.
3. Press into the prepared loaf pan and place in freezer to firm.

Method Top Layer

1. Finely grate the ginger.

2. In a small saucepan place the coconut oil, almond butter, lemon juice and ginger and mix well let it simmer just for a minute.

3. Take off the heat and add sweetener and continue mixing, it will get a bit firmer and kind of make a ball.

4. Squish the topping evenly on the base.

5. Sprinkle with coconut over the top, or use chopped almonds, if you prefer.

6. Place in fridge until set.

7. Remove and cut into cubes. Enjoy.

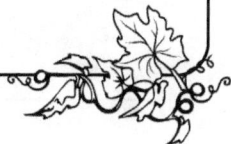

GLOSSARY
OF TERMS

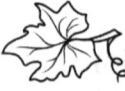

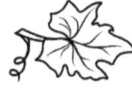

Term	Meaning
Aerobes	Microorganisms which require oxygen to grow.
Achlorhydria	An abnormal condition in which there is an absence of hydrochloric acid secretion in the stomach.
Alpha-sitosterol	A health-promoting cholesterol-like substance which is naturally present in oil-rich plant-based foods, especially some nuts. It is also commonly abbreviated as α-sitosterol in scientific literature. These can be produced by your gut bacteria.
Alkaline	Refers to a pH of over 7 and under 14. From a naturopathic perspective, it also refers to the effect consuming certain plant-based foods has within the body.
Alkalize	From a functional naturopathic medicine perspective, to alkalize means to undertake a nutritional or dietary intervention in order to improve mineral balance within the body. Key alkalizing minerals include calcium, magnesium, potassium and other minerals. To alkalize the body also relates to reducing the acidity of the environment both inside and outside of our body's cells.

Amino acids	These are the building blocks of proteins. There are many different types of amino acids which come from eating a variety of protein-containing foods. There are many different functions and effects amino acids can have in the body. The term amino acid is also shorthand for the longer scientific name α-amino carboxylic acid.
Anaerobes	Microorganisms which require an environment where there is no oxygen present to live.
Anion gap	From a functional naturopathic medicine perspective, the anion gap is a value reflecting the difference between both positively charged ions and negatively charged ions present in the venous blood. See also Chapter 1 for more information.
Autoimmunity	A process whereby the immune cells (immune system) attacks 'self' antigens on healthy cells, tissues, or organs. If such a process is left unresolved, the result can be partial or total cell, tissue or organ destruction and lead to the development of one or more medically diagnosable autoimmune diseases, such as chronic fatigue syndrome, multiple sclerosis, and systemic lupus erythematosus.
Bacteroides	Gram - negative bacteria which require an environment where there is no oxygen present to survive.

Beta-sitosterol	A health-promoting cholesterol-like substance which is naturally present in oil-rich plant-based foods. It is also commonly abbreviated as β-sitosterol in scientific literature. These can be produced by your gut bacteria.
Blastocystis hominis	A tiny single-cell protozoan parasite organism, which is capable of living in the human digestive tract.
Bristol Stool Chart	Also known as the Bristol Stool Scale, is a medical chart that was created by researchers at the University of Bristol (England) in 1997 to help classify stools into seven types.
Chelation Therapy	A type of therapy involving the use of a special substance (called a chelating agent) to bond metal ions, ions or other molecules together so that toxins can be safely removed from the body via the digestive system.
Dientamoeba fragilis	A protozoan parasite that can take up residence in the large intestine of humans and result in an infection.
Dysbiosis	The term used by naturopaths to describe a loss of diversity, or an altered composition, of the populations of microorganisms present in the large intestine.

Endometriosis	Endometriosis is an inflammatory medical condition in which abnormal growth of endometrial tissue occurs outside of the uterus in one or more of the following areas: the fallopian tubes, ovaries or in the tissue lining the pelvis.
Eubacteria	A broad term that means 'true bacteria' and includes most types of bacteria. It includes bacteria which: do and do not have a cell wall (both gram-positive and gram-negative bacteria), lack a membrane-bound nucleus, are single-cell organisms and possess circular DNA which contains a single chromosome.
Fat emulsification	A process occurring in the small intestine during which the surface area of fats from food is increased with the assistance of bile, which has been made by the liver and secreted from the gallbladder.
Fatigue pattern	Refers to the characteristics of fatigue experienced by a patient including fatigue that occurs in a continuous pattern through the course of one or more days, fatigue that occurs at a particular stage of the day over one or more days and fatigue associated with immune compromise or increased susceptibility to opportunistic infections.
Firmicutes	A genus, or group of bacteria most often characterized as gram-positive, which means a thick cell wall structure is present.

Flow Check-up	A key step in Karlene's naturopathic gut protocol geared towards improving digestion and reducing gut symptoms.
Functional GI Disorder	A disorder involving persistent and recurring gastrointestinal symptoms, which are a result of abnormal gastrointestinal tract function. See also: **Rome IV criteria** definition below and in Chapter 1.
GABA	An acronym for gamma aminobutyric acid, which is an amino acid that functions as an inhibitory neurotransmitter in the human brain by selectively inhibiting or preventing some nerve signals in the brain to reduce nervous system activity.
GI	Commonly used medical abbreviation for the word 'gastrointestinal'.
Gram-positive	A term used by microbiologists to refer to bacteria which possess a thick cell wall, as determined by Gram (purple colour based) stain testing.
Gram-negative	A term used by microbiologists to refer to bacteria which possess a thin cell wall, as well as a lipopolysaccharide outer membrane, as determined by Gram (purple colour based) stain testing.
Gut protocol	A rigorous procedure outlining an individualized process for resetting and rebalancing gut health.

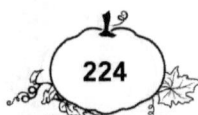

High anion gap	A term referring to acidosis, or higher than normal levels of acid within the body. From a naturopathic perspective, it indicates reduced levels of electrolytes and other minerals for balancing the environment inside and outside of cells within the human body. It can be associated with conditions including impaired digestive function, dehydration, excessive exercise, diarrhea, diabetes or kidney disease.
High Human Intervention food	Refers to the opposite of Low Human Intervention food. High Human Intervention food includes processed and refined food ingredients and food products.
Homeostasis	An innate capacity within a living organism for maintaining and regulating a stable and constant environment within the tissues and cells, which is constantly adapting to influences that are both internal and external to the organism.
Hydrochloric acid (HCl)	An acid which is secreted by parietal cells present within the lining of the human stomach. HCl is an important component of human gastric juices as it helps to break down proteins present in food. It also plays a role in helping to protect the body against parasites and potentially harmful bacteria and viruses.
Hypochlorhydria	A condition in which there is either an insufficiency or a deficiency of hydrochloric acid in the stomach.

Invisible diseases	A variety of autoimmune and inflammatory diseases including multiple sclerosis, arthritis, diabetes, chronic fatigue syndrome, fibromyalgia, mental illnesses and many other diseases.
Insoluble fiber	A type of dietary fiber that includes hemicellulose and cellulose and which does not dissolve in water. Insoluble fiber is present in most types of plant-based foods and is important for good health.
Lipopolysaccharides (LPS)	A pathogenic component, also sometimes described as an endotoxin, which derives from the cell wall of Gram-negative bacteria. This can initiate cytokine release and promote an inflammatory response inside the human body.
Low Human Intervention food	A group of foods including fresh grass-fed, free-range or organic poultry, meat and dairy, as well as fresh seasonal fruit and vegetables, seeds, nuts and gluten-free grains, such as millet, brown rice, amaranth, quinoa, buckwheat, teff and sorghum.
Metabolites	Substances that are either made during, or are required for, metabolic processes involved in human metabolism.
Metabolic Acidosis	Is a condition where there is too much acid being produced in the body. Refer Chapter 1 for more information.

Microbiome	A term including but not limited to the ecological environment and collective genetic material of all microorganisms present within the human digestive tract/intestines. Scientists continue to debate the definition of this term. For further reading see: Berg, G., Rybakova, D., Fischer, D., et al. 2020 in References and Recommended Reading section.
Microbiota	A term that refers to the symbiotic, commensal and pathogenic communities of microorganism located within the human gut/intestines/ digestive system/tract. The microbiota of an individual human being may include archaea, bacteria, fungi, protists and viruses. Scientists continue to debate the definition of this term. For further reading see: Berg, G., Rybakova, D., Fischer, D., et al. 2020 in References and Recommended Reading section.
Overgrowth (bacteria)	An excessive increase in one or more bacterial populations in any section of the digestive tract, including within the gut, the upper digestive tract, and/or the lower digestive tract.
Parasites	An organism that either lives inside of, or on, an organism of another species, which is known as its host. The parasitic organism depends on or benefits from consuming blood, nutrients or some other matter to the detriment of the host.

Perfect poo	A little like Goldilocks! The perfect poo is neither too firm, nor too soft, contains mostly digested food components and is also easily and completely passed via the rectum.
Plant gum	These consist of long chains of sugars, called polysaccharides, which are either contained within foods, food ingredients, food products, or supplements, and are derived from plant-based sources. Gums are capable of absorbing water/are water-soluble.
Pectin	The water-soluble carbohydrate component present in the cell walls and flesh of some fruits and functions to help ripening fruit stay firm.
Polycystic ovaries	A medical condition involving the formation of cysts within the ovaries. Polycystic ovaries (PCO) can be diagnosed by a doctor or other medical specialist after being identified using an ultrasound.
Polycystic ovarian syndrome	A medical condition affecting women of child-bearing age, in which a combination of hormonal imbalance including high levels of androgens, menstrual irregularity and/or polycystic ovaries are present. Polycystic ovarian syndrome (PCOS) is diagnosed in an individual by a doctor according to a defined set of medical criteria and/or a blood test or ultrasound.

Post Protocol Bliss	A good feeling or sensation associated with the experience of ongoing relief from previous gastrointestinal symptoms or other disorders and of optimal digestive function being restored.
Prebiotic	A food component capable of promoting the growth of microorganisms within the human gut.
Probiotic	A living microorganism, which may be present in the form of food or a supplement, which possesses attributes making it potentially beneficial within the human gut for promoting health.
Rome IV criteria	A medical tool used for classifying a set of disorders, based upon gastrointestinal symptoms, including: pain (visceral hypersensitivity), motility disturbance, altered gut microbiota, altered mucosal and immune function, and altered central nervous system processing. See also Chapter 1 for further reading.
Soluble fiber	A variety of fiber which attracts water and is capable of increasing the water holding capacity of the stool during lower digestive tract processes.
Stool	Medical term for faeces. Other synonyms used in this book include: 'poo', 'bowel movement' and 'shit'.

Sweet spot	An optimum combination of qualities or factors to create the most favourable situation possible. In this book, it especially relates to promoting optimal digestive function and gut health.
Your WHY	This is your purpose. Your why is the key to your inspiration and motivation to create the change you seek, and so whenever you find yourself being pulled back to old habits – focussing on your why will help you stay on your new path.

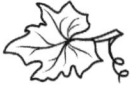

APPENDIX 1

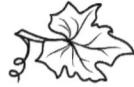

Know Your Shit: instructions for recording your daily symptom chart and poo report

Sign/Symptom	What is it like for me?	Your rating
Digestive – wind, bloating, burping and reflux	The average person farts 4-15 times per day, (the average is 8). Maybe that's spread throughout the day, or maybe you do that over 10 minutes. Windy symptoms are a sign that something is fermenting, and it is time to address what is causing this.	Most signs and symptoms can be rated from 1 to 10. A rating of 1 means the sign or symptoms is minor or rarely an issue, and 10 means the sign or symptom is major or frequently an issue.

Pain pattern and rating	Pain is different for everyone. Where is your pain located? Maybe it is felt in your muscles, organs, joints, or all over your body. What does it feel like? Maybe it is throbbing, stabbing, aching, sharp, or dull. Does it stay in one place, or does it move around? Is it present all the time, or does it come and go depending on the time of day or the time of the month? What is the intensity and does the intensity vary, or does it stay the same?	
Poo	Refer to the stool chart, and remember the optimal poo is number 4 on the chart. Is your stool difficult or easy to pass? How long does it take to pass it? Is there a sensation of feeling the stool has passed completely, or is there still a sensation of fullness? What is the shape? What is the color? Does it sink, or does it float? Do you notice any smell, and if there is a smell, how would you describe the smell?	Please rate the appearance of your stool using the numbers according to the stool chart (rate your stool a number between 1 and 7). Remember, you want to aim for a number four poo!

Energy levels	Perhaps you experience fatigue. If you experience fatigue, does your fatigue have one of the following patterns: continuous or recurring fatigue experienced over the course of one or more days each month, fatigue which reoccurs at a particular time of day, fatigue after food or after the absence of food, fatigue associated with stress, constant fatigue, fatigue associated with immune compromise or an increased susceptibility to opportunistic infections?	
Skin	Perhaps your skin has acne, a rash/hives, redness, itching, or it appears pale or 'off-color'?	
Cognitive function	Perhaps you experience forgetfulness, difficulty remembering information, brain fog, poor concentration or drowsiness?	
Mood	Maybe your mood changes quickly, or doesn't change much at all? Perhaps you regularly experience anxiety, anger, low mood/sadness or other negative emotions?	

Sleep	What is your sleep like? How many hours? What time do you go to bed? How long does it take for you to fall asleep? How many times do you wake during the night? What time do you get up and start your day? Do you wake feeling refreshed, or unrefreshed?	
Immune	Perhaps you seem to catch every bug that is going around, or never seem to get sick at all? How many times have you had a cold or flu in the previous 12 months? How long does it usually take for you to recover? Is it less than a week, or longer than one week? Do stubborn symptoms seem to linger, or do you completely recover?	
Sex and hormonal health	This can include difficulty conceiving, infertility, reduced libido, sexual dysfunction and menstrual cycle irregularities and anything else that is an important sign or symptom for you, so include it here.	

| Other | Is there another important symptom that hasn't already been covered, but is important to you? Perhaps you think it's weird and want to pretend it doesn't exist, but it is real for you? Don't discount it, include it here. It may just hold the key to unravelling your own unique health mystery! | |

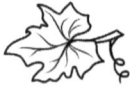

APPENDIX II

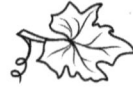

Know Your Shit: your daily symptom chart and poo rating report

Sign/Symptom	What to expect	Your rating
Wind, bloating, burping and reflux		
Pain pattern		
Poo		
Energy levels		
Skin		
Cognitive function		

Mood		
Sleep		
Immune		
Sex and hormonal health		
Other		

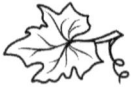

APPENDIX III

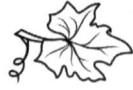

In search of the sweet spot: additional resources

The following lists of food groups relating to histamine, soluble fiber, insoluble fiber and FODMAPs are provided for educational purposes only. When creating each individualised gut protocol, there are many considerations I take into account. The sweet spot for each individual food can vary considerably from one person to the next and as already explained will depend upon the composition of each individual person's microbiota based upon their stool test results. Remember to get tested and work with a practitioner.

Histamine foods to avoid if allergies are present

Here is a simplified list of foods with a medium or high histamine content and are best avoided if allergies are an issue.

Fermented Foods

- All fermented foods and sauces
- Buttermilk
- Kefir
- Miso – all varieties
- Sauerkraut and all fermented vegetables
- Soy – all soy products including tofu, tempeh, soy sauce, tamari
- Yoghurt

Fruit

- Avocado
- Banana
- Berries – all fresh and dried varieties including cranberries
- Citrus
- Pineapple
- Tomato

Herbs/Spices

- Cloves
- Cinnamon
- Nutmeg

Meat, Poultry and Seafood Products

- Aged meats, e.g., beef and pork
- Cheese – all hard yellow varieties
- Chicken liver
- Deli meat – including all processed meat
- Fish – all except fresh caught and gutted varieties
- Shellfish

Other

- Beer/champagne
- Chocolate and cacao
- Sulphites e.g., 220
- Wine
- Yeast

Vegetables/Plant-based Foods

- All red beans
- All red vegetables
- Eggplant
- Sauerkraut and all fermented vegetables
- Spinach

Vegetables and foods high in soluble fiber (excluding fruit)

Here is a list of foods that are high in soluble fiber:

Vegetables
- Avocado flesh
- Beetroot (peeled)
- Brussel sprouts
- Carrots (peeled)
- Collard greens
- Celery (very well de-strung)
- Cucumber (peeled)
- Okra
- Pumpkin (peeled)
- Sweet potato (peeled)
- Turnip (peeled)
- Zucchini (peeled)

Grains
- Oats (can contain gluten)
- Barley (contains gluten)

Nuts
- Hazelnuts

Beans and Legumes
- Black beans
- Edamame
- Kidney beans
- Lima beans
- Navy beans
- Peas
- Pinto beans

Seeds/Seed Husks
- Sunflower seeds
- Flaxseeds
- Psyllium husks

Vegetables and foods high in insoluble fiber (excluding fruit)

Here is a list of foods that are high in insoluble fiber:

Grains
- Brown rice
- Oat bran (can contain gluten)
- Rice bran
- Buckwheat
- Quinoa

Nuts
- Almonds
- Walnuts

Seeds
- Chia seeds
- Pumpkin seeds
- Sesame seeds

Vegetables and Legumes
- Asparagus
- Broccoli
- Chickpeas
- Corn
- Eggplant
- Green beans
- Kale
- Cabbage
- Cauliflower
- Lentils
- Spinach

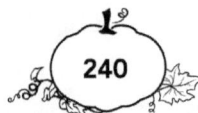

A start-up list of FODMAP vegetables to limit

Here is an alphabetically ordered list of foods that are best avoided or best consumed in limited amounts/serving sizes according to the Monash University low FODMAP diet.

- Artichoke
- Asparagus
- Baked beans
- Beetroot (fresh)
- Black eyed beans
- Broad beans
- Butter beans
- Cassava
- Cauliflower
- Celery – greater than 5cm of stalk
- Choko
- Felafel
- Fermented cabbage, e.g., sauerkraut
- Garlic – avoid entirely – substitute with hing/ asafoetida powder, or garlic oil
- Garlic salt, garlic powder – also avoid entirely
- Haricot beans
- Kidney beans
- Lima beans
- Leek bulb
- Mung beans
- Mushrooms
- Onions, onion powder and pickled onions – avoid entirely
- Pickled vegetables
- Red kidney beans
- Savoy cabbage – over ½ a cup
- Scallions
- Shallots
- Soy/soya beans
- Split peas
- Spring onions – avoid bulb (white part)
- Sugar snap peas
- Taro

*More information about IBS and the Monash University low FODMAP diet can be found here:
https://www.monashfodmap.com/about-fodmap-and-ibs/

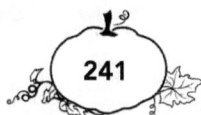

REFERENCES AND RECOMMENDED READING

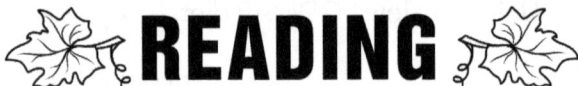

Journal articles

Ahmed, T. and Haboubi, N. (2010). "Assessment and management of nutrition in older people and its importance to health." *Clinical Interventions in Ageing*, 5: 207-16.

Alcock, J., Carlo, C., Maley, C. and Aktipis, C.A. (2014). "Is eating behaviour manipulated by the gastrointestinal microbiota? Evolutionary pressures and potential mechanisms." *Bioessays*, 36(10): 940-9.

Alcock, J., Maley, C.C. and Aktipis, C.A. *"Is Eating Behaviour Manipulated by the Gastrointestinal Microbiota? Evolutionary Pressures and Potential Mechanisms." Bioessays* (2014) 36 (10): 940-49.

Allen, A., Cunliffe, W.J., Pearson, J.P., Sellers, L.A. and Ward, R. (1984). "Studies on gastrointestinal mucous." *Scandinavian Journal of Gastroenterology*, 93: 101-13.

Armstrong, H., Mander, I., Zhang, Z., Armstrong, D. and Wine, E. (2021). "Not all fibers are born equal; variable response to dietary fiber subtypes in IBD." *Frontiers in Paediatrics*.

Becker, D.J. and Lowe, J.B. (2003). "Fucose: biosynthesis and biological function in mammals." *Glycobiology*, 13(7): 41R-53R.

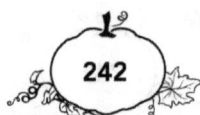

Berg, G., Rybakova, D., Fischer, F., Cernava, T., Vergès, M-CC., Charles, T., Eversole, K., Kinkel, L., Wagner, M., Sessitsch, A. and Schloter, M. (2020). "Correction to: microbiome definition revisited: old concepts and new challenges." *Microbiome*, 8(1): 119.

Buddington, R.K., Williams, C.H., Chen, S.C. and Witherly, S.A. (1996). "Dietary supplement of neosugar alters the faecal flora and decreases activities of some reductive enzymes in human subjects." *American Journal of Clinical Nutrition*, 63(5): 709-16.

Buenrostro, J.L. and Kratzer, F.H. (1983). "Effect of Lactobacillus inoculation and antibiotic feeding of chickens on availability of dietary biotin." *Poultry Science*, 62(10): 2022-9.

Burg, A.W. and Brown, G.M. (1968). "The biosynthesis of folic acid. 8. Purification and properties of the enzyme that catalyses the production of formate from carbon atom 8 of guanosine triphosphate." *Journal of Biological Chemistry*, 243(9): 2349-58.

Caldarini, M.I., Pons, S., D'Agostino, D., DePaula, J.A., Greco, G., Negri, G., Ascione, A., Bustos, D. (1996). "Abnormal fecal flora in a patient with short bowel syndrome. An in vitro study on effect of pH on D-lactic acid production." *Digestive Diseases and Science*, 41(8): 1649-52.

Campbell. A.W. (2014). "Autoimmunity in the gut." *Autoimmune Diseases*, 152428.

Carvalho N.M de., Costa E.M., Silva S., Pimentel L., Fernandes T.H. and Pintado M.E. (2018). "Fermented Foods and Beverages in Human Diet and Their Influence on Gut Microbiota and Health." *Fermentation*, 4(4): 90.

Chen, Q., Chen, O., Martins, I.M., Hou, H., Zhao, X., Blumberg, J.B. and Li, B. (2017). "Collagen peptides ameliorate intestinal epithelia barrier dysfunction in immunostimulatory Caco-2 cell monolayers via enhancing tight junctions." *Food and Function*, 8(3): 1144-51.

Cukrowska, B., Lodlnová-Zádnlková, R., Enders, C., Sonnenborn, U., Schulze, J., and Tlaskalová-Hogenová, H. (2002). "Specific proliferative and antibody responses of premature infants to intestinal colonization with non-pathogenic probiotic E. coli strain Nissle 1917." *Scandinavian Journal of Immunology*, 55(2): 204-9.

Dent, J., El-Serag, H.B., Wallander, M.A. and Johansson, S. 'Epidemiology of gastro-oesophageal reflux disease: A systematic review. *Gut*, (2005) 54: 710-17.

Desai, M.S., Seekatz, A.M., Koropatkin, N.M., Kamada, N., Hickey, C.A., Wolter, M., Pudlo, N.A., Kitamoto, S., Terrapon, N., Muller, A., Young, V.B., Henrissat, B., Wilmes, O., Stappenbeck, T.S., Núñez, G. and Martens E.C. (2017). "A dietary fiber-deprived gut microbiota degrades the colonic mucus barrier and enhances pathogen susceptibility." *Cell*, 167(5): 1339-53.

Dosselaere, F. and Vanderleyden, J. (2001). "A metabolic node in action: chorismite-utilizing enzymes in microorganisms." *Critical Reviews in Microbiology*, 27(2): 75-131.

Ebringer, A. (1989). "The relationship between Klebsiella infection and ankylosing spondylitis." *Baillieres Clinical Rheumatology*, 3(2): 321-38.

Edwards, C.A., Duerden, B.I. and Read, N.W. (1985). "The effects of pH on colonic bacteria grown in continuous culture." *Journal of Medical Microbiology*, 19(2): 169-80.

Gerigk M., Bujnicki, R., Ganpo-Nkwenkwa, E., Bongaerts, J., Sprenger, G. and Takors, R. (2002). "Process control for enhanced L-phenylalanine production using different recombinant Escherichia coli strains." *Biotechnology Bioengineering*, 80(7): 746-54.

Gracey, M., Burke, V., Thomas, J.A. and Stone, D.E. (1975). "Effect of microorganisms isolated from the upper gut of malnourished children on intestinal sugar absorption in vivo." *American Journal of Clinical Nutrition*, 28(8): 841-5.

Grizotte-Lake, M., Zhong, G., Duncan, K., Kirkwood, J., Iver, N., Smolenski, I., Isoherranen, N. and Vaihnava, S. (2018). "Commensals Suppress Intestinal Epithelial Cell Retinoic Acid Synthesis to Regulate Interleukin-22 Activity and Prevent Microbial Dysbiosis." *Immunity*, 49(6): 1103-15.

Guo, L.X., Hong, Y.H., Zhou, Q.Z., Zhu, Q., Xu, X.M. and Wang, H.H. (2018). "Fungus-larva relation in the formation of Cordyceps sinensis as revealed by stable carbon isotope analysis." *Scientific Reports*, 8(1): 5028.

Haan, E., Brown, G., Bankier, A., Mitchell, D., Hunt, S., Blakey, J. and Barnes, G. (1985). "Severe illness caused by the products of bacterial metabolism in a child with a short gut." *European Journal of Paediatrics*, 144(1): 63-5.

Hanh, J., Cook. N.R., Alexander, E.K., Friedman, S., Walter, J., Bubes. V., Kotler, G., Lee, I.M., Manson, J.E. and Costenbader, K.H. (2022). "Vitamin D and marine omega 3 fatty acid supplementation and incident autoimmune disease: VITAL randomized controlled trial." *British Medical Journal*, 376: e066452.

Harmer, C.J., McTavish, S.F., Clark, L., Goodwin, G.M. and Cowen, P.J. (2001). "Tyrosine depletion attenuates dopamine function in healthy volunteers." *Psychopharmacology (Berlin)*, 30(4): 154(1): 105-11.

Hirauchi, K., Sakano, T., Notsumoto, S., Nagaoka, T. and Morimoto, A. (1989). "Measurement of K vitamins in food by high-performance liquid chromatography with fluorometric detection." *Vitamins*, 62: 393-8.

Hockertz, S. (1991). "Immunomodulating effect of killed, apathogenic Escherichia coli, strain Nissle 1917, on the macrophage system." *Arzneimittelforschung*, 41(10): 1108-12.

Hove, H. and Mortensen, P.B. (1995). "Colonic lactate metabolism and D-lactic acidosis." *Digestive Diseases and Science*, 40(2): 320-30.

Jacob, S.E. and James, W.D. (2004). "From road rash to top allergen in a flash: bacitracin." *American Society for Dermatologic Surgery*, 30(4 Pt 1): 521-4.

Ko, T.C., Beauchamp, R.D., Townsend Jr, C.M. and Thompson, J.C. (1993). "Glutamine is essential for epidermal growth factor-stimulated intestinal cell proliferation." *Surgery*, 114(2): 147-53.

Kostiuk, O.P., Chernyshova, L.I. and Slukvin, I.I. (1993). "Protective effect of Lactobacillus acidophilus on development of infection, caused by Klebsiella pneumoniae." [Russian]. *Fiziologicheskii Zhurnal*, 39(4): 62-8.

Kruis, W., Schütz, E., Fric, P., Fixa, B., Judmaier, G. and Stolte, M. (1997). "Double-blind comparison of an oral Escherichia coli preparation and mesalazine in maintaining remission of ulcerative colitis." *Alimentary Pharmacology and Therapeutics*, 11(5): 853-8.

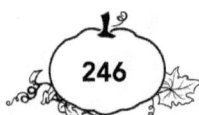

Lee, S.A., Lim, J.Y., Kim, B., Cho, S.J, Kim, N.Y., Kim, O.B. and Kim, Y. (2014). "Comparison of the gut microbiota profile in breast-fed and formula-fed Korean infants using pyrosequencing." *Nutrition Research and Practice*, 9(3): 242-8.

Malchow, H.A. (1997). "Crohn's disease and Escherichia coli. A new approach in therapy to maintain remission of colonic Crohn's disease?" *Journal of Clinical Gastroenterology*, 25(4): 653-8.

Manicassamy, S., Ravindra, S., Deng, J., Olouch, H., Denning, T.L., Kasturi, S.P., Rosenthal, K.M., Evavold, B.D. and Pulendran, B. (2009). "TLR2 dependent induction of vitamin A metabolizing enzymes in dendritic cells promotes T regulatory responses and inhibits T_H-17 mediated autoimmunity." *Nature Medicine*, 15(4): 401-9.

Miller, G.C., Wong, C. and Pollack, A.J. 'Gastro-oesophageal reflux disease (GORD) in Australian general practice patients.' *Australian Family Physician*. (2015) 44 (10): 701-4.

Mulligan, J.H. and Snell, E.E. (1977). "Transport and metabolism of vitamin B6 in lactic acid bacteria." *Journal of Biological Chemistry*, 252(3): 835-9.

Nichols, B.P. and Green, J.M. (1992). "Cloning and sequencing of Escherichia coli ubiC and purification of chorismate lyase." *Journal of Bacteriology*, 174(16): 5309-16.

Oli, M.W., Petschow, B.W. and Buddington, R.K. (1998). "Evaluation of fructooligosaccharide supplementation of oral electrolyte solutions for treatment of diarrhea: recovery of the intestinal bacteria." *Digestive Diseases & Sciences*, 43(1): 138-47.

Pessione, E. (2012). "Lactic acid bacteria contribution to gut microbiota complexity: lights and shadows." *Frontiers in Cellular Infection Microbiology*, 2(86).

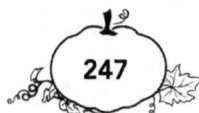

Polen, T., Kramer, M., Bongaerts, J., Wubbolts, M., and Wendisch, V.F., (2005). "The global gene expression response of Escherichia coli to L-phenylalanine." *Journal of Biotechnology*, 115(3): 221-37.

Rembacken, B.J., Snelling, A.M., Hawkey, P.M., Chalmers, D.M. and Axon, A.T. (1999). "Non-pathogenic Escherichia coli versus mesalazine for the treatment of ulcerative colitis: a randomized trial." *Lancet*, 354(9179): 635-9.

Robertson, J., Brydon, W.G., Tadesse, K., Wenham, P., Walls, A. and Eastwood, M.A. (1979). "The effect of raw carrot on serum lipids and colon function." *American Journal of Clinical Nutrition*, 32(9): 1889-92.

Roiser, J.P., McLean, A., Ogilvie, A.D., Blackwell, A.D., Bamber, D.J., Goodyer, I., Jones, P.B. and Sahakian, B.J. (2005). "The subjective and cognitive effects of acute phenylalanine and tyrosine depletion in patients recovered from depression." *Neuropsychopharmacology*, 30(4): 775-85.

Roux, B. and Walsh, C.T. (1993). "p-Aminobenzoate synthesis in Escherichia coli: mutational analysis of three conserved amino acid residues of the aminotransferase PaBa." *Biochemistry*, 32(14): 3763-8.

Salvioli, G., Salati, R., Bondi, M., Fratalocchi, A., Sala, B.M. and Gibertini, A. (1982). "Bile acid transformation by the intestinal flora and cholesterol saturation in bile. Effects of *Streptococcus faecium* administration." *Digestion*, 23(2): 80-8.

Sampson, T.R., Debelius, J.W., Thron, T., Janssen, S., Shastri, G.G., Ilhan, Z.E., Challis, C., Schretter, C.E., Rocha, S., Gradinaru, V., Chesselet, M., Keshavarzian, A., Shannon, K.M., Krajmalnik-Brown, R., Wittung-Stafshede, P., Knight, R. and Mazmanian, S.K. (2016). "Gut microbiota regulate motor deficits and neuroinflammation in a model of Parkinson's Disease." *Cell*, 167(6): 1469-80.

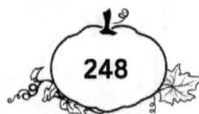

Shah, M., Beuerlein, M. and Danayan, K. (2001). "An approach to the patient with a life-threatening acid-base disturbance: the acidemias." *University of Toronto Medical Journal*, 78(2).

Sivamaruthi, B., Kesika, P. and Chaiyasut, C. (2018). "Toxins in Fermented Foods: Prevalence and Preventions—A Mini Review." *Toxins*, 11(1): 4.

Smith, E.A. and Macfarlane, G.T. (1996). "Studies on amine production in the human colon: enumeration of amine forming bacteria and physiological effects of carbohydrate and pH." *Anaerobe*, 2(5): 285-97.

Smolinska S., Jutel M., Crameri R. and O'Mahony, L. (2013). "Histamine and gut mucosal immune regulation." *Allergy*, 69(3): 273-81.

Soliman, A., De Sanctis, V., Yassin, M., Wagdy, M. and Soliman, N. (2017). "Chronic anaemia and thyroid function. *Acta Biomed*, 88(1): 119-27.

Strandwitz, P. (2019). "Neurotransmitter modulation by the gut microbiota." *Brain Research*, 1693(Pt B): 128-33.

Tiwana, H., Wilson, C., Walmsley, R.S., Wakefield, A.J., Smith, M.S., Cox, N.L., Hudson, M.J. and Ebringer, A. (1997). "Antibody responses to gut bacteria in ankylosing spondylitis, rheumatoid arthritis, Crohn's disease and ulcerative colitis." *Rheumatology International*, 17(1): 11-6.

Tuck C.J., Biesiekierski, J.R., Schmid-Grendelmeier, P. and Pohl D. (2019). "Food Intolerances." *Nutrients*, 11(7): 1684.

Uribarri, J., Oh, M.S. and Carroll, H.J. (1998). "D-lactic acidosis. A review of clinical presentation, biochemical features, and pathophysiologic mechanisms." *Medicine (Baltimore)*, 77(2): 73-82.

van der Wiel-Korstanje, J.A. and Winkler, K.C. (1975). "The faecal flora in ulcerative colitis." *Journal of Medical Microbiology*, 8(4): 491-501.

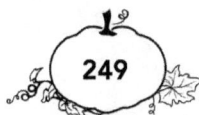

Wallis, A., Ball, M., McKechnie, S., Butt, H., Lewis, D.P. and Bruck, D. (2017). "Examining clinical similarities between myalgic encephalomyelitis/chronic fatigue syndrome and D-lactic acidosis: a systematic review." *Journal of Translational Medicine*, 15(129).

Weltens, N., Zhao, D. and Van Oudenhove, L. (2014). "Where is the comfort in comfort foods? Mechanisms linking fat signaling, reward, and emotion." *Neurogastroenterology and Motility*, 26(3): 303-15.

Williams N.T. (2010). "Probiotics." *American Journal of Health-System Pharmacy*, 67(6): 449-58.

Wu, G.D., Chen, J., Hoffmann, C., Bittinger, K., Chen, Y., Keilbaugh, S.A., Bewtra, M., Knights, D., Walters, W.A., Knight, R., Sinha, R., Gilroy, E., Gupta, K., Baldassano, R., Nessel, L., Li, H., Bushman, F.D. and Lewis, J.D. (2011). "Linking long-term dietary patterns with gut microbial enterotypes." *Science*, 334(6052): 105-8.

Yang, J., Zheng, P., Li, Y., Wu, J., Tan, X., Zhou, J., Sun, Z., Chen, X., Zhang, G., Zhang, H., Huang, Y., Chai, T., Duan, J., Liang, W., Yin, B., Lai, J., Huang, T., Du, Y., Zhang, P., Jiang, J., Xi, C., Wu, L., Lu, J., Mou, T., Xu, Y., Perry, S.W., Wong, M., Licinio, J., Hu, S., Wang, G. and Xie, P. (2020). "Landscapes of bacterial and metabolic signatures and their interaction in major depressive disorders." *Diseases and Disorders*, 6(49).

Yatsunenko, T., Rey, F.E., Manary, M.J., Trehan, I., Dominguez-Bello, M.G., Contreras, M., Magris, M., Hidalgo, G., Baldassano, R.N., Anokhin, A.P., Heath, A.C., Warner, B., Reeder, J., Kuczynski, J., Caporaso, J.G., Lozupone, C.A., Lauber, C., Clemente, J.C., Knights, D., Knight, R. and Gordon, J.I. (2012). "Human gut microbiome viewed across age and geography." *Nature*, 486(7402): 222-7.

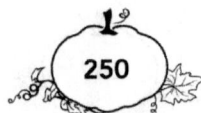

Zhang. X., Rimpiläinen, M., Simelyte, E. and Toivanen, P. (2001). "Characterisation of Eubacterium cell wall: peptidoglycan structure determines arthritogenicity." *Annals of Rheumatic Diseases*, 60(3): 269-74.

Other Recommended Reading

American Academy of Allergy, Asthma and Immunology (2021). "Gastroesophageal Reflux Disease." https://www.aaaai.org/Conditions-Treatments/related-conditions/gastroesophageal-reflux-disease

ATP Science, (2018). "How the gut works in regards to acid and alkali." https://atpscience.com/gut-acid-alkali/

Bagawan, J. (2019). "Babies get critical gut bacteria from their mother at birth, not from placenta, study suggests." https://www.sciencemag.org/news/2019/07/bacteria-free-placentas-suggest-babies-pick-microbiome-birth

Dix, M. (2019). "What is hypochlorhydria?" *Healthline.* https://www.healthline.com/health/hypochlorhydria

European Society of Neurogastroenterology and Motility, (no date). "Diet and microbiota: The influence of diet on gut microbiota." https://www.gutmicrobiotaforhealth.com/about-gut-microbiota-info/diet-and-gut-microbiota/

Monash University. (2021). "FODMAPs and Irritable Bowel Syndrome." https://www.monashfodmap.com/about-fodmap-and-ibs/

Oke, S. (2013). "What does your horse's stool say?" https://thehorse.com/115367/what-does-your-horses-stool-say/

Stevenson, S. (2021). *Eat Smarter: Use the power of food to reboot your metabolism, upgrade your brain, and transform your life.* Hachette Book Group. https://eatsmarterbook.com/

Varney, J. (2016). "Dietary fiber series – insoluble fiber." *Monash University.* https://www.monashfodmap.com/blog/dietary-fibre-series-insoluble-fibre/

Veitch, J., Hume, C., Timperio, A., Ball, K., Salmon, J. and Crawford, D. (2010). "Mental health and physical activity among adolescents." Centre for Physical Activity and Nutrition Research, Deakin University. https://www.deakin.edu.au/__data/assets/pdf_file/0004/376870/mental-health.pdf

Welcome Trust Sanger Institute. (2019). "Babies' gut bacteria affected by delivery method: Vaginal delivery promotes mother's gut bacteria in babies' gut." *ScienceDaily.* https://www.sciencedaily.com/releases/2019/09/190918131447.htm

World Health Organisation, (2020). "Adolescent mental health." *Fact sheet.* https://www.who.int/news-room/fact-sheets/detail/adolescent-mental-health

Books of inspiration:

Healthy Home Healthy Family by Nicole Bijlsma

The Wahls Protocol Book by Dr Terry Wahls

The Wahls Protocol Cooking for Life by Dr Terry Wahls

Eat Smarter by Shawn Stevenson

Atomic Habits by James Clear

Find your Why by Simon Sinek

Food Mood and the Anxiety Solution by Trudy Scott

First We Make the Beast Beautiful by Sarah Wilson

ACKNOWLEDGEMENTS

With deepest appreciation, I know writing this book would not have been possible without the years of mentoring and education received from **Professor Henry Butt Director of Bioscreen.** For every single stool sample submitted, (and there have been thousands), I have spent 20 minutes discussing all the fine details about each sample with the professor who has challenged me to think more about the gut environment, the behavior of the microbiota and how this affects each patient.

When I add these hours together, we have literally spent many years discussing other people's poo! Importantly, Henry encouraged me as I interpreted a stool sample, to always think about what can be done to enhance the growth of bacteria to find the balance that would benefit each patient.

Thank you, Henry, for answering my endless questions and setting me on the path of further research.

To Nicole Bijlsma, thank you for taking the time to read my book and provide your insight in the Foreword. I've been so inspired by your work over the years, I can't believe you took the time to read mine.

To **Dr Denis Rebic at Wellmed** for your care and guidance on this path in the very first instance.

To **Dr Fi Lam** at Valla Beach Health who has encouraged my good work in the field and helped me to spread my wings so that I can reach a wider patient base, and for always having my back.

To **Maggie Wilde and the team at Mind Potential Publishing** for seeing that I had something unique to offer and for helping me believe I could actually write a book! Good heavens, who knew? Well, it seems you did. Thank you for believing in me.

To **Kristi Grbin** for all your work and support in helping this project come to life.

To my thousands of patients who invested in me and in doing a stool sample to achieve great results in their health and wellbeing. Thank you for stepping up.

Finally:

To my loving **Dad** for giving me that firm base of support that said, "*Now is the time to do this, Karls.*" Mum said you are "*good value*", Dad. Of course, she was always right. So wise.

To my dearest **Mum,** forever my inspiration. I feel your energy with me every day.

To my darling children **Nathan and Emily**, who literally were there for me every single day without fail.

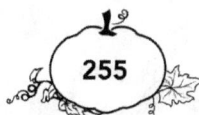

MEET THE
CONTRIBUTOR
NICOLE BIJLSMA

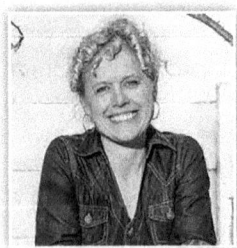

Nicole Bijlsma is a woman of passion, and her passion lies in environmental medicine.

Nicole was a former naturopath and acupuncturist with over 15 years clinical experience who changed her career pathway to become a building biologist after noticing a strong correlation with many of her patients' illnesses and health hazards in their home.

Nicole is the author of the best seller Healthy Home, Healthy Family, and was a columnist for Body + Soul (Herald Sun). She is frequently consulted by the media to comment on health hazards in the built environment (The 7PM project, Sunrise, The Today Show, The Circle, Channel 7 News, Today Tonight, Channel 74, ABC Radio, Fox FM, numerous webinars and podcasts)

Nicole has 30 years experience lecturing at tertiary institutions in nutrition, Chinese Medicine, and environmental medicine, and has published in peer reviewed journals. Her extensive knowledge in environmental medicine has seen her speak at various conferences both in Australia and abroad (USA, Thailand and New Zealand)

Nicole established the Australian College of Environmental Studies in 1999 to educate people about the health hazards in the built environment.

Books by Nicole
Healthy Home, Healthy Family

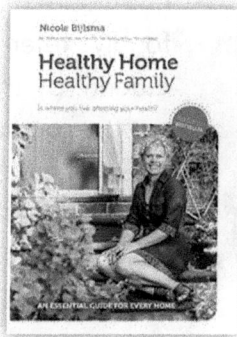

Courses by Nicole

- Create a Healthy Home Course
- Advanced Diploma of Building Biology Certificate IV in Feng Shui
- Mould Testing Course
- Certificate in Electromagnetic Field Testing
- Taking an Environmental Exposure History (for Clinicians)

Website: www.buildingbiology.com.au

MEET THE
AUTHOR - KARLENE
GEORGIADIS

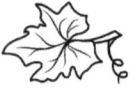

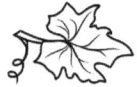

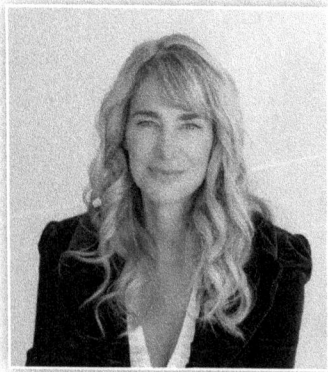

Karlene Georgiadis is a biomedical nutritionist and naturopath and is fondly referred to as 'The Poo Queen' by thousands of dedicated patients and clients. She has literally spent years of her life reading and analyzing other people's poo to understand and solve their greatest health mysteries.

Karlene applies medical pathology testing and scientific research with traditional health principles to uncover and treat the cause of health issues. She then develops personalized treatment plans by interpreting the test results based on the evidence collected from the health data and in consultation with the patient and their symptoms.

Karlene is passionate about being up to date with the latest research and laboratory testing methods.

Who Karlene helps:

- Patients who are sick of feeling like life is a battle and fighting their body and symptoms, just to function normally.

- Patients suffering autoimmune conditions such as Hashimoto's, Chronic Fatigue, Multiple Sclerosis, Diabetes, Parkinson's Disease, Coeliac and Crohn's Disease.

- Patients who are motivated by the accountability and support from a practitioner who cares and is invested in their success.

- People who want to know what it's like to reach optimal health and are prepared to do the work to get there.

Website: www.karlene.com.au

FREE RECIPE BOOKLET

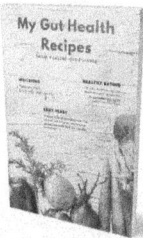

Access a few of my favorite gut health recipes in the bonus chapter of this book. You can also download the complete recipe booklet with many more suggestions by accessing this link: www.book.karlene.com.au/recipes

WHAT OTHERS HAVE TO SAY

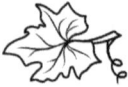

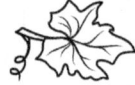

"As a mental health educator, I was very excited to take part in Karlene's Protocol program. The outcomes are amazing especially in relation to my own mental wellbeing. Education has always been an important part of my journey of recovery, and Karlene has been excellent in explaining the causes, and symptoms in assisting me to understand the whys behind the actions of change.

Within one week I started to sleep better, which included no midnight waking. If I do wake now, I go straight back to sleep!

- *My skin has become more youthful in appearance, which is a massive, unexpected plus*

- *My reflux has vanished*

- *I have lost weight and feel less bloated.*

- *I fart less which is a blessing to the whole family!*

- *I have more energy for daily exercise.*

- *MOST importantly - there has been a significant reduction in my levels of anxiety and I not only feel more peaceful but have a clarity of mind that has allowed me to make work and life balance decisions for the good of self and family."*

Jules Haddock- Mental Health Educator

"Thank you for helping me improve my health out of sight this year. PS hot flushes are gone – Yeah!" – Judy

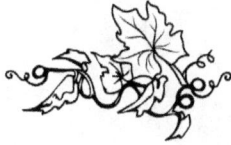

"I cannot thank you enough! You have literally changed my world! I haven't felt this good in a long time. I am so grateful for working with you." – JM

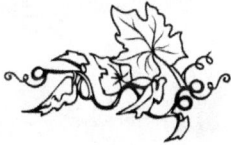

"Thank you for supporting me and getting me back to my feminine self again." – DT

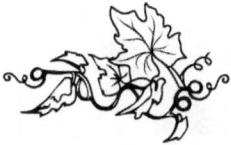

"I can honestly say I wouldn't be where I am or be the person I am, without all of your guidance and support, which I so do appreciate." – MM